Counter-Time

This book explores how trauma affects our experience of time, how that experience may not be linear, and how we may experience "counter-time" – a disruption or arrest of time's flow and a perpetual return to the time of trauma.

Counter-Time explores this phenomenon in clinical practice and in examples from literature and history, including mass trauma such as genocide. Survivors of trauma can be helped to move beyond their experience by drawing on their own cultural resources, helping them to use "counter-time" as a means of release instead of a repeated traumatic symptom.

With rich clinical detail and clear, accessible writing, this book is essential reading for all psychoanalysts and psychotherapists working with trauma.

Marina Breccia is a psychiatrist and training psychoanalyst at the Italian Psychoanalytical Society (SPI) and International Psychoanalytical Association. She is also an external Professor of Psychiatry at Pisa University and foreign consultant for *Revue Belge de Psychanalyse*. She has written several monographs and contributed to jointly authored volumes.

THE NEW LIBRARY OF PSYCHOANALYSIS

General Editor: Anne Patterson

The *New Library of Psychoanalysis* is published by Routledge Mental Health in association with the *Institute of Psychoanalysis*, London.

The purpose of the book series is:

- to advance and disseminate ideas in psychoanalysis amongst those working in psychoanalysis, psychotherapy and related fields
- to facilitate a greater and more widespread appreciation of psychoanalysis in the general book-reading public
- to provide a forum for increasing mutual understanding between psychoanalysts and those in other disciplines
- to facilitate communication between different traditions and cultures within psychoanalysis, making some of the work of continental and other non-English speaking analysts more readily available to English-speaking readers, and increasing the interchange of ideas between British and American analysts.

The *New Library of Psychoanalysis* published its first book in 1987 under the editorship of David Tuckett, who was followed by Elizabeth Bott Spillius, Susan Budd, Dana Birksted-Breen and Alessandra Lemma. The Editors, including the current Editor, Anne Patterson, have been assisted by a considerable number of Associate Editors and readers from a range of countries and psychoanalytic traditions. The present Associate Editors are Susanne Calice, Katalin Lanczi and Anna Streeruwitz.

Under the guidance of Foreign Rights Editors, a considerable number of the *New Library* books have been published abroad, particularly in Brazil, Germany, France, Italy, Peru, Spain and Japan. The *New Library of Psychoanalysis* has also translated and published several books by continental psychoanalysts and plans to continue the policy of publishing books that express as clearly as possible a variety of psychoanalytic points of view. The *New Library of Psychoanalysis* has published books representing all three schools of thought in British psychoanalysis, including a particularly important work edited by Pearl King and Riccardo Steiner, *The Freud–Klein Controversies 1941–45*, expounding the intellectual and organisational controversies that developed in the British Psychoanalytical Society between Kleinian, Viennese and "middle group" analysts during the Second World War.

The *New Library of Psychoanalysis* aims for excellence in psychoanalytic publishing. Submitted manuscripts are rigorously peer-reviewed in order to ensure high standards of scholarship, clinical communications, and writing.

For a full list of all the titles in the *New Library of Psychoanalysis* main series as well as both the *New Library of Psychoanalysis* "Teaching Series" and "Beyond the Couch" subseries, please visit the Routledge website.

Counter-Time

Temporality of Thought and History in Clinical Practice and Literature

Marina Breccia

Translated by Adam Elgar

Routledge
Taylor & Francis Group
NEW YORK AND LONDON

Designed cover image: Alamy

First English edition published 2027
by Routledge
605 Third Avenue, New York, NY 10158

and by Routledge
4 Park Square, Milton Park, Abingdon, Oxon, OX14 4RN

Routledge is an imprint of the Taylor & Francis Group, an informa business

Original title: Contro-tempo. La temporalità del pensiero e della storia nella clinica e nella letteratura

First Italian edition published by Mimesis Edizioni 2022

ISBN: 9781041256281 (hbk)
ISBN: 9781041135135 (pbk)
ISBN: 9781003747581 (ebk)

DOI: 10.4324/9781003747581

Typeset in Bembo
by Newgen Publishing UK

Contents

Acknowledgements

I wish to thank Margherita Giani for her strong support and Stefano Carrara, who has been alongside me reading the text, always devoting an idea of his own to it.

My thanks to Adam Elgar, who has translated the text in a meticulous, profound, and creative way that I have found very valuable.

I also want to remember Adamo Vergine, Valeria Egidi Morpurgo, and Gianluigi Monniello, with whom I would have addressed many of these ideas if only "time" had allowed it. And with them I remember Arrigo Stara, a dear friend as passionate about literature as about psychoanalysis.

Lastly I want to remember the newborn, in the hope that our efforts may be concentrated on "their time" to come; all refugees and their stories of "suspended times"; and all beaten-down and terrified humanity, so that their constructive energies may be harvested in a future time.

Preface

Chiara Saraceno

Entering into a relationship with a text which, for all its generous multidisciplinary openness is rightly, I would say necessarily, a psychoanalytic text, is not only difficult but risky for someone who is not a psychoanalyst. The risk is of talking nonsense or trivialising the subject, or both. And yet I cannot decline to answer the questions which Marina Breccia posed by offering me her book to read: is a cooperative encounter possible in our reading of phenomena, one that may be something more than a simple coincidence between the topics we address or a cross-reference in a footnote? This cooperation is a possibility that Marina Breccia has detected in my work. And indeed, many of the themes addressed in this book also provoke a sociological reflection: the complex and not exclusively linear temporality of experience, the multidimensionality of identity, the struggles of mourning and the difficulty of acknowledging a space for it in contemporary societies so that it can be worked through. In these brief reflections I will dwell on the first two because those are the ones I have found myself dealing with over the course of my research, especially in connection with the transformations in female lives and identities.

The time we experience is not linear

In talking about counter-time as a metaphor both for the experience of trauma and for the analysis that accompanies its solution, Marina Breccia emphasises two different dimensions: that of the arrest, or drag, which stops someone moving forwards or overcoming the obstacle or fracture which has been produced in their life story; and the absolutely dynamic counter-time of contraposition, a different temporality which imposes or facilitates the shift that is necessary for working-through, and hence for regaining a path that can no longer be the same.

But isn't this precisely what is meant by the human condition?

As has been observed especially by scholars who address the whole span of life rather than studying "phases" or looking for rules about passing from one phase to another, the life course is the combined outcome of the bundle of socially and historically situated trajectories[1] in which everyone is inserted at birth or encounters gradually: as son/daughter, brother/sister, spouse/partner, parent, and so on. These multiple trajectories have their own internal interval markers but, as they intersect, they are also to a greater or lesser extent interdependent, prompting accelerations, decelerations, and deviations into one or more other trajectories. The parents' separation or one of them dying may leave its stamp not only on the emotional sphere but also on a child's progress at school and/or work. A premature pregnancy may compel the redefinition of plans at work or at home, and so on. Studying the course of female lives, Gerson (*Hard Choices*, 1985) highlighted how life experiences can modify aspirations by shifting investments from one trajectory to another. Disappointments or checks in professional life can make a woman who had initially invested in her professional career re-orient her aspirations and the investments she had put into "success" and the value of the couple relationship and motherhood. Conversely, an unsatisfying or terminated couple relationship may mobilise investments and capacities in a professional sphere which had initially not been considered as something worth achieving. Or again, the experience of success, or simple satisfaction and the perception of one's own value in the professional sphere may stimulate interest in a career for a woman who had initially considered it marginal to a way of life mostly oriented towards investment in her family.

In other words, even when one has a clear idea of what one wants to do in life and makes organised moves in pursuit of it, life can surprise us and compel us to re-orient our goals and investments into one specific trajectory, but also from one trajectory – one dimension of our identity – to another: not only, or necessarily, reductively but also in a facilitating way. It is a thesis which further dynamizes the theories about psychosocial development proposed by Erikson

(1950) and Levinson (1978), for whom the process of arriving at adulthood and then maturity happens through successive phases of constructing an equilibrium between the areas of emotional, cognitive, and relational investment, of crises in this equilibrium and the construction of a new one. The approach to life introduces into this dynamism of various successive, more or less orderly phases in reorganisation of the self, the possibility of unexpected disruptions, deviations, or impediments. In this context, Smelser ("Issues in the study of work and love in adulthood", in N.J. Smelser and E.H. Erikson, *Themes of Work and Love in Adulthood*, 1980) holds that any formulation of a theory about the course of life should contain at least four ingredients:

a) a statement of the continuous and repeated *challenges* to a person over the life course, both anticipated and unanticipated;
b) a statement of the *resources* available to the individual who faces this array of challenges;
c) a statement of the *adaptive responses* that take place when life-course challenges and individual resources confront one another in concrete situations;
d) a statement of the *historical accumulation* of a person's responses and orientations, in that the life course can be regarded as an accumulation of historical precipitates of the challenges one confronts and the resources one brings to meet those challenges.

None of which involves a judgement about whether this accumulation should be understood as maturation, growth – or, on the contrary, decline – or a mixture of all these. Pearlin too ("Discontinuities in the study of aging," in T. Hareven (ed.), *Transitions: The Family and the Life Course in Historical Perspective*, 1982, and "Life strains and psychological distress among adults," in N.J. Smelser and E.H. Erikson, op. cit.), critiquing the linear and orderly view of the life course proposed by many theories of development (which, not by chance, talk about "phases of the life cycle"), maintains that it is not necessarily the events and transitions considered most important – normative – by society which produce the greatest stress or the perception of a radical change, or even the perception of a radical change on the part of the person experiencing it. Rather, it is "anomalous," unexpected events. While expected events prompt anticipatory adaptations (which therefore happen over a longer, subterranean span of time), unexpected ones can require adaptations and reorganisations for which there are no rules or anticipated socialisation.

"Theorists of the life course" also place the accent on another aspect. Interference does not only happen between the trajectories on which each of us has set out. It may also happen between the life courses of closely linked people. This is the phenomenon which Elder and Moen have called *linked lives*.[2] What happens in the life – professional, health, emotional – of one's partner, parent or child may have an impact on the decisions we make about our own life. Here too, female life stories are the most obvious example since their choices and the experiences to which they are exposed, even in their own homes, are often determined by what happens in their partners' professional trajectories,[3] or by the care needs that arise in their family network as their parents age or grandchildren arrive. But the phenomenon of linked lives may express itself in an apparently more nuanced though equally powerful way in less obvious or less normative contexts too. Some years ago, during an investigation into female life courses, I interviewed a very busy professional woman who had given birth to twins and so was reorganising her commitments, which included negotiating timings and responsibilities with her equally busy husband. During the interview it emerged that although the two children had arrived unexpectedly, they were the result of a much wished-for pregnancy which had happened sooner than the couple had originally planned. In fact, the decision to have a child had been brought forward when the woman's father was diagnosed with a terminal illness which left him with little more than a year to live. So the woman, and the couple, had wanted to give the father a chance of fulfilling his desire to be a grandfather. His illness had produced a profound transformation in the lives of at least five other people: his wife, daughter, and son-in-law, and the twins (who otherwise would not have come into the world when they did). I have met grandmothers who have retired early to help a working daughter with childcare, elderly couples who have moved house and changed the setting of their lives and relationships, so as to live near their sons and daughters and help with the grandchildren (but I have also known sons and daughters who have gone to live as far as possible from their parents, in order to add physical distance when relations are difficult).

So perhaps counter-time is the prevailing temporal rhythm of many life courses whose seeming linearity is more the outcome of a self-representation than censorship or a reformulation of the interruptions, deviations, and re-thinkings as if they were intentional, leaving no residues. As John Lennon sang in *Beautiful Boy*, "Before you cross the street/Take my hand/Life is what happens to you/While you're busy making other plans." Trauma, and then the time of analysis, are probably its extreme expression: the former as an interruption that blocks, an impasse as Marina Breccia rightly calls it, instead of the opening-up of a different possibility; the second as its necessary working-through because a counter-time, even when dramatic and negative, does not block the possibility of retaking control of one's own life story, taking it on and narrating it (to oneself), and so also enabling it (and oneself) to explore and seize the possibilities of moving on. But how many people, even without having undergone particular traumas, remain blocked by a failure of their ambitions, by the perception of an injustice suffered, or a decision that did not have the desired outcome? And they live facing backwards, regretting (sometimes rancorously) what they might have been, what they might have done "if only," and thereby close off other paths, other desires for themselves.

Dynamic and multidimensional identities

The multiplicity of trajectories that compose a life course suggests that everyone's identity consists of a plurality of dimensions which are added to, or lost (though leaving traces), or assume greater or lesser significance over a lifetime. Personal identity is the composite and dynamic outcome of this multiplicity of dimensions, of facets, as Marina Breccia writes in the chapter devoted to heterogeneous identities:

> So a re-reading of the Freudian corpus may leave us to consider identity as a sort of historical memory of the various configurations that the Ego has assumed through perception of the experiences with the objects in which it is identified and the outside world. It is an Ego operating within the single individual and that precise subject in relation to the history that concerns it, *its* history, and thus to all the parental models that have preceded it and lie deposited transgenerationally in its identity-forming experience.

> These deposits accompany the many early investments deposited in objects.

And she goes on,

> It is thus by virtue of this plasticity of the mind, in continuous and lively motion by means of its re-combinatory capacities, that the features which contribute to the identity are sufficiently multiple and heterogenous, from the archaic residues to the combining and re-combining with experiences deriving from current relationships and the re-actualising of relationships, as in the transference.

The conception of the life course as a bundle of trajectories (situated historically and culturally) and relations allows us to see identity as a complex and dynamic construction, hence mutable over the course of a life story. This mutability not only concerns the process of growth and aging, but also the encounter, more or less peaceful or conflicted, with the socially normed and/or accessible identity models relating to gender, sexuality, couple relationships, motherhood or fatherhood, social class, religion, ethnicity, work, and so on.

The awareness that the individual is the outcome of a multiplicity, a plurality, is greater in some societies which we consider backward because they lack the typically Western concept of a person as a compact and indivisible unit.

As Remotti shows, along with other anthropologists before him, in many African cultures it is taken for granted that the person is a "we" which can be decomposed and recomposed on the basis of relationships and experiences. This is why anthropologists propose the term "dividual" in place of "individual" (Remotti, *Contro l'identità* [Against identity], 2001). According to Remotti, thinking about the persona as plural by no means prevents us seeing its uniqueness, which is fully enabled by its unrepeatability. The specific combination of dimensions and relations of which every person is composed is in fact unique and unrepeatable.

And yet the question of the plurality and dynamicity of identity was addressed by Giddens (*The Transformations of Intimacy*, 1992) as if it were a specific trait of contemporary developed countries where the plurality of positions that a person occupies simultaneously and the multiplicity of experiences they can have over the course of a life – and thus the possibility of changing them – are greater than in the past, making it difficult for anyone to imagine themselves (and represent themselves to themselves) as identical and immutable both in the relational space and in time. According to Giddens, in this situation identity can only be reflexive, the outcome of a constant process of self-reflexivity.

Plural or reflexive identity does not mean that, depending on the phases or circumstances of life, one aspect of the identity, one relationship, one trajectory, cannot weigh more heavily than the others and in some way also determine them, or be privileged in the public representation of oneself. When Giorgia Meloni says, "I am a woman, I am a mother, I am a Christian," she is choosing a representation of herself which apparently overshadows the dimension of her identity as the leader of a political party on the Right in favour of what nevertheless has temporal priority over the other facets of her identity. Choosing to foreground those dimensions of one's identity may be instrumental in some cases while in others it may answer to the personal system of priorities at that moment and in that context; in yet others it may (also) have a self-protective and reassuring function. Some years ago an American sociologist (whose name I have unfortunately forgotten) researching women with careers was astonished to note that their first act in the interview was to present themselves as mothers, as if to conjure away the suspicion that their having a career made them seem less like women and, God forbid, inadequate mothers. Because each of us, in defining our own identity, must take account of the expectations and generic definitions evoked in other people and laid down in the process of socialisation by one of our group characteristics – in this case, being women. Conversely, the strong presence of a father in childcare may be perceived as risky for self-presentation in a context where this scenario could be regarded as weakening the masculine identity (to the point where in Italy it may be labelled with the somewhat disparaging term *mammo*) and professional reliability. It gives pause for thought that there are Italian fathers who, in order not to risk being perceived as unreliable by their employer, and despite having the right to days, or at least half days, of parental leave, prefer to use their holiday allowance if they are at home with a sick child.

As Marina Breccia also reminds us, group identities can have a totalising ("tyrannical") – I would say all-consuming – effect on other, more personal dimensions of the identity, especially if they are those of a minority or a group who, even though they are a numerical majority like women, are nevertheless a minority on the plane of symbolic and social power. They may have this effect on the way they see and classify us, and open or close opportunities to others – others such as women, Black people, Jews, Muslims, migrants, homosexuals, transsexuals, and so on and so on – resulting in varying degrees of depersonalisation.

Nevertheless, the same individuals may have recourse to more or less temporarily and completely totalising group identities: to mobilise around discriminations considered unjust; to make visible and thus to legitimate socially the group they belong to; to exclude others;[4] or even to justify personal choices or failures – or not face them.

Oscillating between group identities and a personal – multidimensional – identity, and even playing around with these different dimensions, is a common experience. It is when group identity – but I would also say a single dimension of identity – absorbs everything without leaving room for distance, comparison, reflexivity, reducing the individual to a single dimension and a single trajectory to be followed, that the game becomes dangerous: for oneself and, in some cases, for others.

Notes

1 Cf. Elder, 1984, 1994, 2000.

2 Cf. Elder, 1994, 2000; Moen, 2003; Moen et al., 1995; Bengston et al., 2005; Settersen, 2015.

3 Until 1968, when an important judgment by the Court of Cassation ruled that it was unlawful, in the light of the constitutional principle of equality, that women in Italy were obliged to move house if their husband's work or other interests required it, or else be charged with abandoning the marital home. In fact, the civil code, not yet reformed at that time, stipulated that the wife must follow her husband wherever he decided to set up home.

4 Remotti's reflections in *Contro l'identità* are to a large extent devoted to collective identities constructed as totalising and "pure", and their intentionally or *de facto* exclusionary function.

Introduction

Trauma is a topic which often fascinated Freud, as it did many early psychoanalysts. It has been much used, sometimes inflated, sometimes over-simplified, just as the criticisms of its complexity have sometimes been over-simplified and trivialised.

Nevertheless, I am aware that it remains an inexhaustible subject and I wanted to examine the subtle and intricate conceptual web that radiates from it, using as my starting point a concept of temporality characterised as *opposition to time*, hence the book's title.

This opposition to time involves an opposition to advancing, to going beyond, to re-establishing a continuity with life, and hence with death; an opposition that may consequently result in a death with no end and thus with no conclusion. So, death accompanies many chapters of this book: psychoanalytically theorised as the death instinct, destructiveness and mourning, as well as the concept of psychic reality which aligns with a historical existential reality in its religious, anthropological, literary, and biological permutations, following a process that aims to psychicise the historical and historicise the psychic. The diffusions of trauma as a central theme have in this way found further possibilities for extension and dialogue. Mourning, for example – the arduous human effort of recomposition, as many historical, religious, and anthropological sources confirm – was frequently addressed by Freud. Indeed, the work of mourning, like that of dreaming, represents humankind's unrenounceable attempt to leave the darkness behind and restart a living temporality that will have an *end* (as purpose) and an *end* (as termination). The purpose is argued over by the many identitary

DOI: 10.4324/9781003747581-1

aspects which inhabit us, and those human beings who would rather ignore this inescapable multiplicity battle madly and blindly with each other to the point of annihilation.

Unfolding an extensive network of subjects in a dialogue between disciplines has inevitably been a complex project. I have found it very helpful to keep asking myself about the motivation behind it and how it could be realised, since it is a project where extension is constantly faced with limits and boundaries. And so, what I *meant* to write and what it *means* to the reader as we set out into the territory of other disciplines, much-loved by me though not practised, are the products of a passionate search for a possible dialogue; an interior, private dialogue inside the writer, but not without intense conflicts.

Counter-time in music is *counterpoint*, inserting a voice into the fundamental cantus which enters on and accentuates not the downbeats of the bar but the upbeats, making a rhythmic contrast with the other voices.

In music, *syncopation* and *counterpoint* are phenomena linked to rhythm, with the intention of producing variety in the unfolding of a passage. More precisely, *syncopation* is the production of *sounds* corresponding to the weak accents of a bar (the upbeats), which are protracted into the next sound. The effect of this is a temporary suspension of the natural metre imposed at the start of the musical passage, creating greater movement than in a perfectly matched musical argument. Syncopation thus imposes a shift of the rhythmic accent from the strong (down) beat to the weak (up) beat, a sound that starts on the weak beat and is prolonged onto the strong beat, weakening accents that would have been rhythmically strong and strengthening those accents that would have been rhythmically weak. Counterpoint provokes a similar effect to syncopation with the difference that, in this case, instead of notes on the weak accents of the bar, the *pauses* occupy the accents of the strong beats, leaving the notes with the space that corresponds to the weak beats. There is extraordinary early evidence of the art of syncopation and counterpoint in the Mediaeval *Hoquetus* and it finds later superlative examples in the compositional virtuosity of Bach's fugues and, to cite only a couple of masterly illustrations from classical music, in the works of Scarlatti, especially the harpsichord sonatas, and in the third variation of Beethoven's sonata no. 32, op. 111. There is also a reinvention of cross-rhythms at the heart of African music which, nearer to our time, finds its way into swing, a structural rhythmic feature of jazz and jazz-inspired improvisation.

Suspension and temporal delay, shifting from strong to weak beats, counterpoise, heterogeneity, crossings: all of these are strong symbolic elements, transposable to the contents of trauma and to the way they operate in clinical work, their irruption into a session, and the analyst's engagement with it all. Perhaps there is nothing in analytic work comparable to Bach's fugues, but there certainly is a correspondingly great capacity for listening to traumatic counter-time, since it is the small variation that indicates the change within the repetition, and it is this temporal opposition which becomes the element that safeguards a future temporal movement so that it may recover its vital rhythms.

A collection of reproaches and small checks, left deposited for several years, have brought to life the many versions of a trauma and the need to rework it clinically as well as the need for the many intersections involved in autobiographical writing: a temporal multiplicity is the distinguishing feature of both. I would add that this is the same temporal multiplicity which accompanies the developmental and processual phases of the identity-forming structures and their transgenerationality, of which traces remain in great traumas such as genocides – first and foremost, the *Shoah* – and in the long periods of latency that are needed for them to emerge. We also encounter this long latency in very different clinical situations such as the "psychotic potential" which needs a great deal of time and several generations to reveal its underlying secret and to defuse the bomb that accompanies it.

How difficult can it be to defuse "in time" the intention to enact the temporal end of life and convert the traumatic experience from tragic to conflictual? These experiences are to be discovered, grasped, maintained in their difficult and precarious dynamicity.

And so, step by step, the hints that preceded the text have also generated it, linking up together within it and gradually extinguishing their singularity by leaving space and time for a reticular unity that is more suffered: whole and yet unfinished, in constant competition with loss and mourning. Stories are presented in sessions, challenging linear temporality, not so much in the way they move towards re-signification *a posteriori*, *après-coup*, but rather through a temporal subversion, a stalemate and a confrontation with time, all of which evoke the traumatic situations that are being recounted. I have wondered if this rhythmic challenge only applied to the contents or also to my relationship with them, to my history in rhythmic contrast with the other histories. It is not the obvious answer to say it could hardly be otherwise, since the aspect that is not obvious lies in exactly this interplay, which naturally remains beneath the surface.

As in musical and choral counterpoint, the contents of this volume, though divided into separate chapters, also inevitably intertwine with one another, breaking the soloistic rhythm and forcing it firmly backwards, in a way that does not defeat the rhythm, but simply stands against it. However, this is only one of the temporal pluralities to which the title alludes, since my writing has tried to track a variety of times – historical, psychic, biological, poetic, literary, artistic: both linear and decomposed, dislocated times, with new harmonics, and with their synchronies and diachronies, and the infinite range of possibilities for revisiting them.

As I was writing the book I too encountered a counter-temporal impasse: Covid-19, a large-scale traumatic event, global in extent and thus defined as a pandemic, which inserted itself as a potent COUNTER-time into the already challenged time of writing. And in a sort of *telescopage* – to recall Piera Aulagnier, who will feature repeatedly in this volume – it sometimes happened during the writing that one thing slipped into another, coming into it from outside, slowing thought down and at the same time stimulating and enriching it. I decided to deal with it as it presented itself, as an interference that I should modulate myself into without being carried away or deported; in fact, much more time needs to be spent thinking back on all this than I spent on writing the book.

I called this moment an *impasse*, naturally with reference to my personal experience of life and writing because I felt the coming of Covid-19 as an explosion in a succession of great traumas that were colliding with history at that moment. The social reaction was a total convergence on the epidemic, in an assertive or negationist manner, and an ignoring – in some cases an annulment – of any attention to, interest in, and above all, any anxiety about the rest: a sort of massive, global, yet obscure counterinvestment. I believe the most significant impact and impasse derived from this second human response rather than from the nevertheless pervasive, tragic nature of the first. Growing societal hatred, out of proportion to growing inequalities and ever-increasing poverty and economic crisis, already far advanced before Covid and, with them, other human baggage such as racism and anti-Semitism, anti-Islamism and hostility to religion in general,[1] xenophobia, homophobia, persecution and exploitation, terrorism, kidnappings, wars, and the still unchallenged arms trade have continued to worsen unabated, ignored by a humanity almost anaesthetised by the pandemic. These extensive phenomena which were once called "mass" and now, in an apparent extension of perspective, are called "global," continue their onward flow, just as in recent decades other great traumas, more silenced, more circumscribed but no less extensive, have recorded increases which have likewise been obscured, despite having afflicted history for a long time, such as sexual abuses (inside and outside families), violence against women or their degradation, and the state of submission imposed by fundamentalist theocratic regimes.

While my mind was looking for a way of organising the writing that would *bring time* to these events and reconstruct them as history, as well as analysing the predominant traumatic function of opposition to time, of going counter-time, and while I was looking for analogies and correspondences with the great collective traumas of the past, the Covid event imposed itself, and in turn counter-imposed itself, with its own historical and global traumatic charge, though it too was not without precedent and analogies in history.

And all the while, in a clamorous silence, a matricidal-suicidal war has been raging, one of the greatest that history has known, and perhaps entirely unprecedented: that of Humankind against Nature. It has been going on without a trace like an apparently silent guerrilla, shrouded in a quasi-mafioso silence, under the cover of mad economic justifications, or sometimes signalled as an exceptional event, fruit of malpractice and viewed with resignation in the face of human error like the nuclear disaster at Chernobyl in 1986 which, as Ukrainian obstetricians can testify, is still causing birth defects today, or the 2011 nuclear disaster at Fukushima Dai-ichi in Ōkuma. Even while dying, Nature has been rebelling against global warming, bringing floods, desertification, hunger, failed harvests, deaths, and mass exoduses equal to those caused by wars, in one long interminable journey. Without an adequate and responsible capacity for understanding, Humanity has been giving paradoxical responses, pitting man against man, naturally the more fortunate against the deprived, a behaviour which was regrettably reproduced even by some governments during Covid.

This was happening yet again as a repetition of one trauma flowing into another, with an ever more blocked, sometimes counterpointed temporality as if breaking a rhythm that has taken a fearful course, leading to the most recent sudden slide into the pandemic.

Words are trying to use this excessive burden as a starting point, trying to join up with each other and with others outside the text.

The extension of this blocked time into slippage from trauma to trauma, blocked likewise from the future, led me – as I have already recalled – to a comparison with other disciplines, to represent the features of this extension by adopting other viewpoints, in the Socratic spirit of one who seeks knowledge, who aims to fill the gaps in what they know and to enrich themselves with other people's knowledge. The intention was nevertheless to draw from these encounters the strength to go ahead by thinking psychoanalytically, stimulated by newly opening scenarios, new surprising and unexpected perspectives, sometimes being proved seriously wrong as well as finding incomparable and comforting astonishments. This strength corresponds to a principle which I find ever more convincing: the principle that we do not save ourselves on our own, and that the more dramatic and traumatic the event, the more ridiculous, wretched, even destructive it is to boast of one's own knowledge. Both the past and the present have often borne witness to this wretchedness.

This model of knowledge is certainly not new or original and has sometimes been unfairly scorned by disciplinary individualisms and exclusivity, and by conformism generally. However, I am convinced it is a model of knowledge that will be indispensable for future generations as the surest antidote to the risk of a single dominant mode of thought.

The heterogeneous multiplicity of the comparison between disciplines is matched by a heterogeneity of readers to whom this volume is addressed. Psychoanalytic thought is always there as a background trace but sometimes it becomes an emergent trace which assumes communicative characteristics more specifically directed towards transmission, while at other times it is more submerged as a background that enquires with my interlocutors into several themes – historical, literary, artistic, religious – or current events. This has perhaps been the most difficult part of the journey: maintaining the specific focus of my language when addressing these latter themes while sacrificing some of the features more associated with technique so as to foster a more extended conversation. The aim of all this has not been to dilute or to popularise but to open an internal dialogue directed towards comparison.

Einstein liked to recall that he got on so well with Freud because one of them knew nothing about psychoanalysis while the other knew nothing of physics, but he also liked to emphasise that when the most complex thing is clear in your mind you can explain it to your grandmother. It could be said of him that he was a man in constant movement between *heimlich* and *unheimlich*, the familiar and the uncanny, the alien: a movement and search that I would wish for the generations to come.

Perhaps the experience that is gradually growing year on year makes us more inclined to address younger readers and talk to young people enriched by other experiences of learning and by the exchange with other, international cultural spheres, in the hope that we may begin a search as a group, perhaps as a collective, for a way to save a common cultural good and a renewed desire to increase it productively. Because, as Arrigo Stara[2] often used to remind us, culture is the only common heritage that matters; and he said this in the hope that younger generations are not afraid to draw on the past, a past that symbolically refers us back to our origins, so that they can acquire indispensable knowledge and build the future. Much of this is the domain of psychoanalysis, as Nathalie Zaltzman recalled in 2007, recognising that psychoanalysis is a *Kulturarbeit*, work for the sake of civilisation.

However, I also felt the desire to address the less young, my own age group, those who have at least partly shared this experience, and those who have helped me to orient and manage it in life, in the consulting room, and in my research. I wish to express my thanks to this last group, a gratitude that, even when reciprocated, is inevitably close to nostalgia, a nostalgia caused by separations, expressions of a vital demand that achieves autonomy and in separating does not divide, and thus allows rediscoveries to be made even from astronomical distances. As Freud said, the object is not found but always re-found.

In the end one is still writing a story, using a subterranean story of one's own, a life story from the future, and the writing is inevitably also infused as much with its subject matter as is it with this slippage of thought which re-encounters returning elements in the different chapters in a sort of structural recursion.

The first chapter enters the twilight zone of the interdisciplinarity which accompanies the whole voyage with varying degrees of salience. The second chapter is devoted to trauma and its temporal and counter-temporal complexities, and links not only with the intractability of clinical journeys – sometimes under baking sun through arid, sandy canyons; sometimes in frozen ascents on menacing escarpments; and sometimes over murky, stagnant, muddy waters – but also with the analyst's inner crossings. The analyst who pictures these scenarios along the way, reactivating and capturing some of their elements in the transference, tries to foster the other person's capacity for configuring them so they can then have the satisfaction of discovering that these elements are completely different from what they had tacitly imagined. And so, areas of shadow and stalemate enter into counter-time. Time sometimes seems to break: that aspect of the subject which is *counter-poised* against time, as it is imagined flowing, is imposed on the object. Humankind's fears of the present and the past meet in the third chapter, devoted to rituals and repetitions. The fourth chapter is again concerned with present time and with the current moment, a time exposed to action and hence counterpoised against thinkability. In that chapter metapsychological contents come together with other elements drawn from the historical and social reality of the present, with its worrying and tumultuous upheavals resulting in the dramatic experience of identity being negated, with its complex and no less dramatic reactive solutions. A chapter, the fifth, is devoted to genocide and the *Shoah* in particular, since genocides have been – and, as we must painfully remember, still are – the unforgettable historical testimony to a dislocation and upheaval of identities resulting from the oppression of one social group by another in an intolerance of such diversity which reaches the point of physical annihilation. This is a collective trauma with specific characteristics both in the possibility for the victims to work through it and in the transgenerational trace that remains deposited in future generations and can only sometimes be expressed after very long periods of latency. Writing has been a form of testament for many victims of genocide, but also for others who, though not having been persecuted, have wanted to bear witness. Writing and in particular biographical writing is the subject of the sixth chapter. The topic has been chosen to emphasise the complexity of the traumatic *re-crossing* that writing offers to both writer and reader. If all writing is also inevitably autobiographical, this feature does not in itself define the libidinal investment of the object which it may represent and propose, because it may instead just be the hypostatic testimony of a past that is no longer alive, one with no "filial" urge to be remembered. Or else writing may, on the contrary, become a legacy with a desire to be transmitted, shot through with loss and mourning, a legacy which takes it upon itself to hand a responsible reworking of that past over to the future. It is precisely this more or less lengthy *crossing-time* which leads to the reflections and topics of the seventh chapter, in which the definition *crossing-time* – i.e., passing actively through time – has been chosen in preference to *time passing* – i.e., a mere interval of time, an interval which every crossing imposes and brings into existence. The chapter is especially devoted to that difficult time-crossing that may be encountered in clinical work and is necessary for lighting up a possible path towards treatment of *psychotic potential*, a theoretical-clinical theory of Piera Aulagnier, to whose ideas a part of the same chapter is devoted. The eighth chapter offers various interpretations of the term *end*, together with the theoretical and methodological complexity of treatment in situations where the urge to end life engages the analyst professionally and personally on several fronts. And it is by virtue of this engagement that the chapter is interwoven with the epistolary philosophical-literary text by Rousseau, *Julie: or the New Héloise*, to show how the analyst's attention and interest turn to the states of conflict evoked by the theme of life's conclusion rather than to the threat of a conclusion in the form of a drama, a threat which nevertheless looms over the consulting room and risks compromising the analytic work on it.

It is a story which seems long even in summary, like a long walk through mountains which reveals ancient places rendered new by their rediscovery and opens up unexpected scenarios which, without the partial perceptual isolation of writing, would perhaps remain impenetrable.

"The time is out of joint" Shakespeare, *Hamlet* (Act I, scene v).

Notes

1 These expressions of hostility to all forms of religion are ever more widespread in the Western world, in parallel with an apparent countertendency manifested by certain strongly nationalistic governments who use religions for political ends, turning them into

an ideological banner and an instrument of propaganda. These last uses of religion, though very unlike those in Middle Eastern theocratic regimes, maintain a veil of ambiguity over religions and a potential distortion of their history and meaning.

2 Arrigo Stara was a man of letters, teacher of Theories, Forms and Institutions of Contemporary Literature at the University of Pisa. For the "Meridiani" series published by Mondadori he edited *Tutte le poesie* (1988) and *Tutte le prose* (2001) of Umberto Saba.

I

THE SHADOW ZONE

In a book where many topics revolve around trauma and its temporal intricacies, I find it essential to recall the aspect of theories that is traumatic because of their revelatory potential, and equally essential to offer a reflection on what I call the *shadow zone of theories*.

Theories cannot flow into each other or be blended; they cannot colonise other theories or be colonised by them. Theory can be considered an abstraction derived from a representation of experience which would in itself be too fragmentary and incomplete, and yet theory metaphorizes it, making no claim to replace it but instead trying to meet the need to render experience thinkable. Gaps between theories are therefore inevitable, and not only for historical or scientific reasons, but because in psychoanalysis they are used to plumb the unconscious parts which gave them the impulse to emerge.

So I find that the attempt to resolve the conflicts between different analytic theories, along with the search for "invariants" – common, shared elements – seems to risk creating further conflicts since the invariants that are indispensable for one theory may not be for another. This does not mean ending up in a disastrous relativism, or a postmodern scepticism often characterised by a loss of faith in the progress of humanity (Lyotard, 1979).[1] I am clearly not taking a relativistic view of individual knowledge: on the contrary, I am thinking about a cooperative conflict between theories, since I am convinced of the need for a new cooperation for the future

DOI: 10.4324/9781003747581-2

of psychoanalysis. I have borrowed the term "cooperative conflict" from the economist and philosopher Amartya Sen, who won the Nobel prize for economics in 1998 and currently teaches at Harvard, focusing his studies on economic ethics. In *Development as Freedom* (2001) in particular he argues for a paradoxical relationship between efficiency and individual freedom which, in my opinion, resonates strongly with disillusionment about our power to overcome conflicts without surrendering to an inconclusive relativism, but also accepts imperfection as inevitable, indeed indispensable. For this reason, some opponents have accused him of individualism.

Amartya Sen warns us against groups that are sectarian instead of cooperative: the danger, as he sees it, lies in defending the values of an identity with an ideological blindness which constructs identities that kill. In support of his thesis Sen does not only draw on the science of economics but also draws a map of examples taken from history. These aspects will be extended and developed in Chapter IV, "Present and Current/Actual: Multiple and heterogeneous identity – identity denied."

I am inclined to see in his work not only a complete anticipation of our current historical and societal condition, but also an effective prompt for reflecting psychoanalytically about a comparison between different theories.

There is no guarantee against such a comparison being put to dogmatic use. Nevertheless it is surprising how few obstacles stand in the way of a slippage in that direction. I believe that as analysts we should maintain the model advised by Freud in *Analysis Terminable and Interminable* (1937) and engage in a continual comparison of theories. Freud alerts us to the possibility of unlimited analysis: "The business of the analysis is to secure the best possible psychological conditions for the functions of the ego; with that it has discharged its task" (p. 249). If this is where it reaches its limits, it cannot and must not do otherwise. But for this very reason Freud calls upon analysts to test themselves constantly against other sources of verification.[2]

However, I find it not only necessary to make these checks against the psychoanalytic theory that we take on board because it suits us best, but also with theories from outside our discipline, since it is in the gap, in what confounds expert thought, that we find a renewed and transformed opportunity to think and rethink.

Using a botanical metaphor, I would like to recall that there are plants that cooperate with each other and some that do not. For example, in the phylogenesis of oaks it has been hypothesised that forest fires have paradoxically fostered their conservation because they need to stand apart from each other or else they die in the shade of trees too close to them. However, other plants have a vital need for cooperation: beech trees with pines and spruce, for example. Beeches grow in clearings among pines because they need the pines' shade.

Psychoanalysis too needs the shade of other disciplines, just as do psychoanalysts themselves. It is curious that the phrase *shadow zone*, like *twilight zone* or *grey area*, has strong connotations of narcissism, a narcissism of death. Conversely, I believe that *the shadow zone* is what stops thought becoming stereotypical, whatever form it takes, from the sacred to the ideological. The logic of the oak tree is not at all dialectical but committed to surviving at other plants' expense, even those like itself, waiting for external destructive events to help it survive.

Freud's interest in Anatole France's *La révolte des anges* of 1914, written at the start of the First World War, is no surprise, and not only because of Freud's many literary interests, but also because of his attentiveness to the social and political debates of the time, debates in which France took part as a novelist, poet, and journalist. With Zola he defended Dreyfus and won the Nobel prize for literature in 1921. In his novel *The Revolt of the Angels* France builds the plot around two parallel figures, a bourgeois who wants to live a tranquil life of indifference, disengagement, and privacy, and a rebel angel preparing a new assault on heaven. Of course, the metaphorical implications cannot have failed to strike Freud, and their foresightedness still strikes us today, anticipating the Second World War and, we could add, the wars of our own time, as well as the pandemic, all characterised by individualism and lack of responsibility. But Anatole France's metaphor is also a helpful warning to any extended, societal group functioning where indifference and glib bullying superficiality create opportunities for tragic upheavals. So Freud's warning seems to put analysts on guard, especially in their clinical work, to ensure they keep themselves open to what I like to call the shadow zone.

This zone is also what delimits an approximate band of terrain within which seismic phenomena are not visible to survey stations: sadly and inevitably, every station has one, and only cooperation between several stations enables adequate coverage in monitoring the earth's surface.

The shadow zone is also what Conrad describes in his novel *The Shadow Line* as the difficult, threatening, potentially deadly region, the place where an illusory youth is abandoned.

The shadow zone is also a border region, a border that may become a cut, a splitting of the subject from their identity, as clinical work testifies. On the subject of separation-splitting, Michael de M'Uzan says in *Aux confins de l'identité* [At the boundaries of identity] (2005),

> In fact, what is meant by separation has not acquired unanimous meanings: it can refer to an experience of a phenomenon or a process [... and] it bears two strictly opposite definitions: on the one hand it can be understood in terms of cutting and dissociation, while on the other it refers to differentiation and distinctness. Then again... it is an intrapsychic phenomenon and so, when one speaks of separation from the object, one is talking about a separation from an invested representation or from a perceptual trace. It is important to be precise about this because such a representation is not only the object of a libidinal investment but, through being located within the psychic apparatus, it is also the object of a narcissistic investment.[3]
>
> (2005, 124–125)[4]

In a psychoanalytic context, the shadow zone is the zone of absence which requires a cooperative function: the possibility of representing absence, i.e., of transforming the intrusive trace of absence.[5] So this possibility is not a premiss but the outcome of a dialectical process. The intruder can be killed by a passion, the affective passion that every idea may bring with it, made for clutching onto a single immutable and indissoluble identity, exhaustive in itself and hence never heterogeneous.

Shadow, this physical phenomenon by which a body interposing itself between a surface and a light source projects "its own" dark area on the surface, stirred the imagination of artists such as Caravaggio and poets such as Dante, Shakespeare, and countless others in an extraordinary heterogeneity of representational possibilities. The shadow zone of theories serves to indicate both their encounter with each other – possible and necessary even though they may be in conflict – and their boundaries and inevitable limits.

Notes

1 Lyotard, 1979, *The Postmodern Condition: A Report on Knowledge.* There the author treats the postmodern as the end of modernity and as a critique of the grand metaphysical narratives of all the idealism and ideology that determined a social cohesion in modernity, fostering a Utopian revolutionary but totalising impulse. According to Lyotard, this decline opened up a search for non-universal judgements and legitimisations. To me it seems possible to link this with Freud's structural model and its introduction of the death instinct, though we should recall that in *Civilisation and Its Discontents* (1929) Freud took a longer view, oscillating between faith in progress and disillusionment about the ethical possibilities of an advance in civilisation.

2 Freud, 1937, *Analysis Terminable and Interminable* (p. 249): "It seems that a number of analysts learn to make use of defensive mechanisms which allow them to divert the implications and demands of analysis from themselves (probably by directing them on to other people), so that they themselves remain as they are and are able to withdraw from the critical and corrective influence of analysis. Such an event may justify the words of the writer who warns us that when a man is endowed with power it is hard for him not to misuse it.... [A footnote refers to Anatole France, *La révolte des anges*.] Every analyst should periodically – at intervals of five years or so – submit himself to analysis once more, without feeling ashamed of taking this step."

3 [Translator's note: the quoted passage is translated from the author's own Italian version of the French original.]

4 Another link with Chapter IV.

5 I think it is clear from what I have said about the shadow zone, as I call it, that this is different from the theoretical concept of the *shadow* proposed by Jung, a concept that undergoes evolutions-variations as that author's theory develops, following the historical perspective of his thinking, but which I nevertheless think it is important to recall. Indeed, for Jung *shadow* initially had a psychological meaning, referring to the deeper part of the personality (*Psychology of the Unconscious*, 1912–1942), and later took on a supra-personal and supra-temporal dimension until it acquired the status of an archetype.

II

TIME IN TRAUMA

It was undoubtedly an initial reflection on trauma and its complex temporal characteristics that animated the thinking which resulted in this book. Much has been written about trauma and it can sometimes seem as if everything has already been said, and that even the critiques of what has been written may fall into the repetitive reductionism they contest.

In the end, as Bollas has characteristically reminded us, dealing with trauma is traumatic and thus exposed to the risk of repetition, or at least to the threat of ending up recycling the evidence, as it were, in an attempt to convince oneself of what one thought already: a reassurance and defence against the threats of an unknown that is more disturbing than any other.

This chapter centres mainly on the less evident aspects of temporality in trauma and on their possible meanings, but also considers how to position oneself in this temporality; the kinds of complexity the analytic work may encounter compared to work in apparently less traumatic clinical situations, at least in terms of the treatment offered; how much this temporality is inevitably impregnated with action and its defectiveness in terms of symbolisation; and how thinking and analytic work may find ways to bring all this to a representational transformation and a transformative representability.

DOI: 10.4324/9781003747581-3

The fixed and repetitive temporality of trauma is also undoubtedly entangled – and sometimes arrested to the point where the instincts become blocked – with a *historical* temporality, that of each subject's individual history in which the trauma has been located, bursting into their story, throwing forward movement into confusion, leaving sometimes distorted and misleading traces of a linearity, always assuming that individual non-traumatic historical journeys do exist and that linearity can easily be rediscovered in a non-traumatic situation. In addition to taking up a position in the trauma, looking for paths towards symbolisation and thinking, psychoanalytic work has the aim of regathering the scattered threads of history, a history sometimes reduced to scraps, clearing a possible path even where there seem to be insurmountable chasms in the way. Repression has failed and it makes little sense relying on a return of the repressed to build historic bridges with the past when the past is missing. Sometimes the past must be constructed before being reconstructed, and this sort of historical prosthesis is not simply a completion or the satisfying of an idealising order free of conflicts. On the contrary, it is deeply meaningful, setting in motion and bringing new sense to the time that was stalled by the intrusion of the traumatic experience and the consequent impossibility of transforming it. In the end this is the essential psychic characteristic of trauma: the impossibility of transformatively *re-signifying* the traumatic event.

So, historical-temporal construction and re-connotation in the psychoanalytic process take on the characteristics of a subjectivity that recounts its life story as it is being reconstructed and, in doing so, presents itself with a gift of sense and meaning as a legacy that reconnects with a past while at the same time being an investment in the future. Patients often do not know they are patients because they do not even know who they are as subjects, and this gives us the measure of the pioneering undertaking they are sometimes engaging in with us psychoanalysts.

Some literary narratives will help me along the way, and I will accompany them with case histories that do not correspond exactly with extracts from clinical work but inevitably draw on my clinical experience of trauma. This decision is not only designed to protect the privacy of individual patients but also has the function of confirming the autobiographical character of writing, a characteristic I have tried to address at greater length in Chapter VII. Although this is a complex aim, it does not overlook the necessary persistence of the scientific endeavour that underpins it, since it is this endeavour which supports the technical, methodological, and theoretical hypotheses built up through clinical experience and proposed in the text.

How to make the "evident" temporality of trauma non-evident

Addressing the theme of trauma and its treatment using a psychoanalytic approach means first of all being able to face numerous difficulties concerning theory.

While psychoanalytic theory in its varied theoretical permutations is complex because of the difficulty linked to the psychic phenomena being investigated, a further complexity is added by the fact that the object under investigation is an intrinsic part of the instrument doing the investigating. Perhaps this is the reason why an author of the 1960s, the well-known proponent of a theory of psychosis, Piera Aulagnier, drawing on both the Freudian and Lacanian traditions, alerts us against easy reliance on theory and the psychoanalytic method in this clinical area: "As I proceeded, I realised… that certain questions that I thought had been resolved had become once again obscure, certain concepts that I believed to be no longer problematic had lost their apparent clarity" (1975, p. xxv).[1] I believe that Aulagnier's warning about psychosis can be exported to any clinical situation and could become a motto for psychoanalysis: *Make what appears evident non-evident.*

But after all, isn't this always helpful?

We could consider Aulagnier's theory as a sort of high road which is not a facilitator of thought, as some critiques of psychoanalysis aim to be by offering an alternative to it, claiming that they will reach a wider audience: rather, her theory is a path towards curiosity and libidinal investment in research and study, and aims to prevent the anaesthetic effect caused by easier access to its contents.

What is communicable without reservation, however, is her passion for discovery.

A further intention of this chapter is to suggest some theoretical avenues towards trauma and to highlight their possible relations with and obstacles to the process of phantasying so as to shed light on both the theoretical difficulty of the relationship between trauma and phantasmatic processes and – as I see it – the indispensability of phantasy for clinical work.

I will now set out some reflections on the methodology of the clinical process over the long duration of recovery from trauma. These hypotheses go further than simple waiting, which is justified by the complexity and difficulty of the phenomenon, and I want to place the symptom in a working setting where the analyst is getting to grips with a more specific complexity: that of what happens to the traumatised Ego and what is made possible thanks to the unconscious elements that are evoked by analytic work.

So I will try to analyse the defensive systems of the Ego that has been subjected to trauma, using some general principles but taking the individual variables and the analyst's defensive systems into account. Above all, I will try to explore the conditions for psychic survival by both members of the analytic couple in the long periods spent re-actualising the trauma in the sessions.

Another premiss seems essential with regard to the psychopathological aspects of traumatic experience. There cannot be a psychopathology of trauma *per se* since it is a characteristic process of the human species that crosses the path of the sane subject just as much as it does to a subject already in a pathological situation, putting both at risk. It thus takes on the characteristics of a cross-section, a continuum between pathologies and between pathology and normality. However, I think a distinction also needs to be made between describing the "trauma as a phenomenon" and the metapsychological framework or frameworks that define it, so that we can immediately reveal this double lens – one that distances by way of abstraction and the other that gets close enough to the clinical phenomena – and try to set up some relations between the two. The intertwining of theory and practice is a key element of psychoanalysis, enabling inevitable deviations, new possibilities, new metaphors, and, as Jean-Yves Tamet recalls in "The Emergence of the Object" (paper read at the 82nd Congrès des Psychanalystes de Langue Française, Paris, 2022), psychoanalysis comes up against the "*objeu*," an untranslatable neologism that fuses *objet* (object) and *jeu* (game, play) coined by the poet Francis Ponge in 1961 in *Le soleil placé en abîme*.

The term *trauma*, long used in medicine, derives from the Greek and indicates both the wound and the piercing that causes it. The double definition as active and passive will return as a guiding thread through this account. However, I recall that in a later linguistic turn, the Latin *traumaticus* means a place for accessing a cure, indicating the relationship between the site of the wound and the place which is open to treatment, but also the gateway, the breach, and the possibility of passing through it which, as I feel I must emphasise, is inevitably in two directions.

If Freud is our starting point we must recognise that the economic conception of trauma becomes central and almost absolute in the *Introductory Lectures on Psycho-Analysis* (1916–1917), as he himself affirms when he maintains that "the term 'traumatic' has no other sense than an economic one. We apply it to an experience which within a short period of time presents the mind with an increase of stimulus too powerful to be dealt with or worked off in the normal way, and this must result in permanent disturbances of the manner in which the energy operates" (1917, p. 275). This concept will become fundamental in *Beyond the Pleasure Principle* (1920), where, in support of it, he uses the metaphor of a protective – para-excitatory – layer or "shield against stimuli" which, if torn, leads to trauma because the protection against excessive and thus intolerable stimuli has been reduced. Hence the psyche's defensive functioning which mobilises counterinvestments that may foster the block against the site of the excitations so as to restore a condition that functions according to the pleasure principle.

The economic factor in trauma thus becomes a clear advance on the concept of trauma in the *Studies on Hysteria* and *Draft K* (1895a). Indeed it is well-known that Freud abandoned the *seduction theory* which, besides the element of transgression, implied excitation of the erogenous zones provoked by the adult seducer. This theory made sexual trauma the basis of neurotic disturbance. At the same time Freud was developing theories of the defences, but both concepts – seduction and defences – are constantly evolving in his thought and precise correlations cannot be established between them, even though they can never be separated. In fact, the traumatic event, studied while he was still beginning his theoretical consideration of repression as a defence, is considered traumatic precisely because it prompts this pathological defence. Such was the state of his research at that moment.

I will briefly mention that, according to the well-known evolution of the seduction theory, trauma unfolds at two times separated by puberty: the first, the seduction properly so called, represents an advance by the sexual which finds the child-subject unprepared, and in this phase there is no repression. The second event, which, after puberty, necessarily has a sexual character, re-evokes the first through some associative features. Then, because of its charge of endogenous excitation, the memory is repressed. It will be the return of the repressed that gives meaning to the trauma *après-coup*, and giving meaning also means managing, modifying in the light of subsequent traumatic events.

And so, according to this evolution in the theory, it is not only that the trauma has a deferred effect, but the temporal element, through the numerous possibilities for the return of the repressed, allows unforeseen features of a pathology correlated with it to be seen and discovered.

At this point we should ask ourselves if the consequences are only pathogenic, but at the same time it must be stressed that in the second trauma theory, which is mainly economic in character, repression is bypassed as a defence and from this new viewpoint it is specifically the Ego's difficulty in using repression which characterises the trauma's greater pathogenicity.

Two other lines of thought emerge from this.

The fact that the first event may not be repressed entitles us to speculate that it is not representable: or rather, *that it may not be represented symbolically*, at least with its original intensity.

The other point is that the passivity of the seduction scene *does not only mean that the subject behaves passively*, but also that the scene cannot evoke a response in them: the connection to sexuality will only be made later because at the moment the subject is not ready for it.

I also want to add that this hypothesis of the two times of trauma is highly indicative of the hypothesis which Freud would develop more fully later on, by which *external events draw their efficacy from the "phantasies" they activate and from the afflux of instinctual excitation that they provoke* (see *Project for a Scientific Psychology*, 1895b; *Introductory Lectures on Psycho-Analysis*, 1916–1917), and this is how the flow of the subject's history is kept in contact with psychic reality, just as history itself will help Freud to develop.

In fact, when Freud introduces the economic conception of trauma in 1918, after the end of the First World War, new perspectives open up, offering psychoanalysis new opportunities for comparison because of the *pathologies with which the history of the period is imbued*,[2] as is also demonstrated by the papers read at the Budapest conference of 1918 by Ferenczi, Abraham, Simmel, and Tausk, on "the dreadful devastation that has come over the world" (Tausk, *On the Psychology of the War Deserter*, 1916, p. 356).

While, on the one hand, these contributions give a voice and conviction to psychoanalysis in relation to an exclusively organicist neurology which had been in confrontation with it until that moment, on the other hand they allow a change of position, seriously revisiting the concept of trauma and introducing a marked interest in psychosis, in defences such as splitting and projection, and a recovery of the concept of narcissism. They also turn their attention towards research into the fate of the libido in relation to the aggressive impulse[3] and the outcomes for the Ego.

So in 1920, in *Beyond the Pleasure Principle*, a work in which Freud develops his second drive theory, the economic definition of trauma as wounding and consequent disequilibrium in the psychic economy is reprised, since it determines an enormous afflux of excitation that puts the pleasure principle out of action and compels the whole psyche to give priority to a more urgent task: that of binding the excitations in order to permit a deferred discharge, above all so that it does not devastate the subject. This extension of the theory endows trauma with a far greater valence less restricted to the sexual sphere, though without in any way challenging the seduction theory or the support given in trauma by phantasy. Trauma is not just a disturbance in relation to libido theory but radically threatens the subject's integrity. Hence the further study of the defences and the consequent introduction of the psychic agencies that will form the foundations of the structural model presented in *The Ego and the Id* (1922), as a result of which he will, from now on, talk about Ego defences. The concept of trauma will be taken up again in *Inhibitions, Symptoms and Anxiety* (1926), which endorses a sort of symmetry – and I would say inevitable exchange – between internal danger and external danger, and he hypothesises a *primal trauma* as the origin of the affects and of anxiety. In *Constructions in Analysis* (1937b) Freud finally acknowledges the impossibility of remembering traumas experienced in the earliest stages of life, during the first two years, since they happen before the acquisition of language. Their evocation may then take unexpected forms as hallucinatory states or irrepressible repetitive actions.

So the concept of trauma runs throughout almost all Freud's work and, with encouragement from history, is especially found at an important crossroads in his thought, from which innovations and transformations of his thinking will emerge. We should also ask ourselves if the concept of trauma, besides being a persistent feature of Freud's thought, was also a constant generative spur because of the inevitable contamination-commingling between trauma, history, and drives.

Persistent presence and active generation are always a feature of writing and of any creative work. Thought not yet completely expressed to consciousness, thought seems to guide the hand and, in the act of writing, to anticipate the writer's own consciousness. As should not surprise us at all in a theoretical hypothesis about the drives, Freud at first emphasised how the Ego always comes late to its own experience of itself.

Does the pianist follow his own thought as he plays or is it the playing that guides it?

While the concept of trauma follows almost all of Freud's work under the surface, it also becomes a strong provocation, causing further theoretical and paradigmatic voices to emerge in later thinking, to which I will refer only briefly. Two years after the publication of Freud's *Three Essays on Sexuality* (1905), Karl Abraham[4] stressed that trauma cannot be the cause of hysteria and *dementia praecox* but only the triggering factor in an already predisposed child. (He probably chooses to name these two pathologies to prompt the psychoanalysis of the time into a deeper study of psychosis, as he had done from 1904 to 1907 when he was assistant to Bleuler at the Burghölzli. A little later, in 1910, Freud wrote "The Schreber Case," using the autobiographical material of Daniel Paul Schreber suggested by Jung). In a second work of the same year Abraham talks about the endogenous character of the genesis of trauma: "If there is an underlying unconscious wish for it, the experiencing of a sexual trauma is a masochistic expression of the sexual impulse" (1907, p. 370) and this is why the child feels shame and guilt, which, according to Abraham, are reasons for traumatic suffering. The interesting and controversial aspect of his thinking is the fact that the event is considered immaterial, or only rendered material by unconscious phantasy.

Ferenczi took a different view, shifting the centrality of the problem onto the modes of communication and the capacity (first of the parent-caregiver and then of the analyst) for listening. In this he wishes to show that in neither case is the adequacy of their capacity for listening to be taken for granted. He hypothesises that care and help are missing at the start, when they should in fact be fundamental, and this narcissistic mortification, suffered by the child because of the inadequate response to their needs, is what sustains and maintains the trauma, along with the *acrobatics* which the child must perform in order to adapt to it. Extending the concept of seduction, Ferenczi develops a remarkable theoretical and metapsychological process, proposing that the traumatic aetiology is based on the psychic violation of the child by the adult in what he calls the *confusion of tongues* between baby and adult. According to Ferenczi, the psychic violation is fostered and maintained by the adult's denial of the child's trauma. So what happens is that, in a splitting process, one part of the child's psyche dies, amputated, and the other lives or, we should say, survives, defending itself but in destructive ways and constantly threatening the integrity of the subject, who is consigned to a living death.[5] Therefore (with Otto Rank, 1924) he postulates a *fractured catharsis* which is achieved thanks to the engagement of the analyst who is ready to share the repetition of the trauma and thereby foster the possibility of modifying it in memory. Only by *living* the traumatically interrupted experiences *to the full* (Ferenczi, 1933) in the present interaction with the analyst can the patient arrive at a new solution: this is his theoretical-clinical hypothesis.

So from the start trauma acquires different senses and quite a few points of contrast between one theory and another.

Again briefly, I will also note Kris's "shock trauma" and "strain trauma" (1956, pp. 54–88); Winnicott's (1960) *relative* trauma caused by failure of dependency on the idealised object which becomes hated; the *cumulative* trauma of Masud Khan (1974, pp. 42–59); Sandler's (1997) *retrospective* trauma; and Greenacre's (1967, 1973) *screen memory* which obscures the trauma. We should recall the contribution made by Laplanche to the concept of trauma, considered as a foundational and thus structural aspect of the psyche which leaves untranslatable residues as well as those which can be translated. (I will just mention "Fantasy and the Origins of Sexuality" (1968) written with Pontalis, and the dictionary of Freudian concepts, *The Language of Psycho-Analysis* (Laplanche et al., 1967). On the relationship between trauma and fantasy which recurs throughout this book and its close links to the untranslatable residues just mentioned in Laplanche's thought, see Giaconia and Racalbuto, "Il circolo vizioso trauma-fantasma-trauma" (1997), a work in which the authors pick up Freud's concept of a "foreign body," regarding it as non-mentalisable, and view phantasies as a coherent and circular production, continually self-generating in a vicious circle – a concept of phantasy which thus heightens its degree of untranslatability.) If we look at more recent evolutions of the concept of trauma, Christopher Bollas sees a self-limiting element in trauma because of its life-changing features ("trauma is just that, traumatic," Phillips, *The Christopher Bollas Reader*, 2011, p. 59) and hypothesises that the subject's unconscious may make use of a "receptive" function which enables them to "re-envision" the trauma ("trauma is just that, traumatic," Phillips, *The Christopher Bollas Reader*, 2011, p. 59).

A concept in continual evolution.

By enhancing our thinking with the diversity of views available in the work of other authors, we can recognise that an aspect not completely illuminated by Freud is the weight of influence brought by the Other in organising the temporal dimension of trauma. This binomial – influence of the other/temporal organisation in trauma – fosters and conditions the evolving characteristics of the trauma in various ways with repercussions that are by no means negligible in their impact on psychic life, beginning with the possibility of construction and reconstruction in phantasy. These aspects are much more distinguishable in clinical work.

I will now return to a few passages from Freud's *Beyond the Pleasure Principle* (1920) to introduce some observations about aspects of temporality in trauma in relation to the Ego defences. In the second chapter of this paper Freud investigates the prevalence of the traumatic element over the pleasure principle in dreams and play.

Everyone is familiar with Freud's description of his grandson Ernst's cotton-reel game. The boy was a year and a half old, praised by the servants and his parents for his good nature since he never cried when his mother went away. He had in fact invented a game that he used in situations when his mother was not there: he took a wooden cotton-reel and hurled it under his bed to make it disappear, accompanying this with an expressive "*o-o-o!*" which, according to his governess, stood for "*fort*" (gone), and then making it reappear, saying "*da*" (there) with satisfaction. The game centred on the child's ability to *determine* the object's disappearance and reappearance *repeatedly*, and Freud interprets the active meaning of the game as being to dominate the anxiety caused by his mother's disappearance. It is interesting that in a note (p. 201, n1) Freud adds that Ernst repeated the game with himself, making his reflection disappear and reappear by crouching under a mirror that reached almost to the floor, a fact that must have greatly struck Freud since he added it the same year, 1919, to a new edition of *The Interpretation of Dreams* (1900, p. 461, n1).

However, Freud does not develop the possibility of further relations between trauma and play as a repetitive symptom, even though he was very curious about Ernst's games and the possible relationship between these and some behaviours connected to the traumatic experiences that the boy was going through.

Ernst was the first child of Sophie, Freud's fifth child, born in 1893, who at the age of twenty married a portrait photographer from Hamburg, sharing a tranquil if not luxurious life with him. Sophie died six years after her marriage, immediately after giving birth to her third child, weakened by the Spanish flu. Freud was very close to his daughter and his grandson and perhaps for this reason did not expand his reflections on Ernst's defensive systems in more detail, not feeling absolutely neutral about it. (It is very moving to read the deeply affectionate words in which, writing to Abraham, he describes the way this grandson smiled at him.[6]) We should also ask how far the new theoretical view of trauma drew on the historical reality of that moment which certainly had an impact – the catastrophic outcomes of the First World War followed by the influenza epidemic – and how much of a subterranean autobiographical trace was left by this terrible bereavement (that of surviving one's children), compared to what he had already shown in *Mourning and Melancholia* (1915a).

For example, Freud recalls that while Ernst was very young, the night before his father was due to leave for the front, he had a nightmare in which he called out for his father, sobbing violently. In recalling this, Freud points to a rediscovered confirmation that the dream-work succeeds in transforming the psychic *material* into a wish-fulfilment, whereas the *affect* belonging to it persisted unchanged in sleep. Freud's interpretation of Ernst's nightmare is that Daddy and Baby can thus stay together while the crying continues to acknowledge the imminent separation.

The "long-drawn-out and peculiarly stressed *'o-o-o'* had been one of his first words" a few months earlier when "he had played at 'gone' with all his toys" (*Interpretation of Dreams*, 1900, p. 461, n1, added in 1919). However, on that occasion, the throwing of toys went in only one direction, as a *gone* with no return, like the "Go to the front!" (1920, p. 16) angrily addressed to his father. It was a separation impregnated with a great deal of destructive rage, a throwing-away for good, a condemnation imposed on another so as not to suffer it oneself. Perhaps Ernst found more egoic control of the object in the cotton-reel game, which would not however save him from the tragic experience of being orphaned while still young.

Freud's description of Ernst's games indicates that his little grandson learns to differentiate powerlessness in the face of danger (evoking the primal anxiety, *Hilflosigkeit*) from the possibility of mastering the danger by anticipating it (the cotton-reel game). He also differentiates the real, foreseeable danger from the instinctual, less foreseeable one.

As I see them, symptom and play have a fundamental value in releasing the Ego from an activating excitation suffered after, and as a result of, the trauma. Through the wounding action coming from outside, passivity, the inability to effect a change in the crushing and distressing experience, in fact mobilised an activating inner excitation both on a purely somatic-instinctual level and on a psychic-phantasmatic level. This activation can, and necessarily does, go on in two directions: on the one hand the activation is devastating in its potential for disorganisation of an already fragile Ego – and the disorganising effect is founded on the continual re-actualisation of the trauma; on the other hand, it is the only resource the Ego possesses for any future psychic reorganisation, and for not feeling totally cast aside by the passive experience.

Using clinical material, I will try to assess the importance of this "binomial" through work done on the elements that have given rise to it.

"*Petrified*"

A number of patients have made me think about aspects of trauma and helped me to recognise that the symptom they use to overcome it presents deeply autobiographical characteristics. These are patients who have never experienced psychosis, although they may have had experiences of splitting. The body is only apparently separate from psychic time: though it is marked by the transformations of age it often preserves the traumatic scars which the mind will later be able to work on autobiographically.

While it is true that any activity of thought, study, or research, but also of historical or speculative "reconstruction," may be understood as autobiographical (as Piera Aulagnier indicated in her interpretation of Freud), this entails complex psychic work, largely submerged because it is unconscious, which takes a variety of forms before emerging as conscious expression. Chapter VI of this book is devoted to this and many other aspects of the autobiographical characteristics of symptoms and writing.

The unconscious autobiographical aspect may introduce its expressions and meanings into the analytic process while the working-through of the trauma is in progress; and so I will try to highlight the movements that the analytic *work* may find itself going through, my aim being to make clear how this is a project of recomposition.

A central difficulty is the question of whether we can entrust this project to a newly emerged *subject* which has only just made itself capable of sustaining and nurturing it. Another difficulty is whether or not we can yet make use of the subject in the processes of recovering and re-signifying subjectivity. Before all this is possible there may be repeated failed attempts to achieve an effective completion, leaving behind traces, fragments or distortions, as would be the case when it is not a pen that is doing the writing, and what is being written on is not a sheet of paper but a body, for example – as has happened with some of my patients – and I have decided to summarise some important clinical features condensed into a single figure.

In the following clinical case history, the play of the narrative is interwoven with elements of reality in an intentionally distorted manner so that the points of contact with reality are lost. The aim is prompted by the hope that the experience emerging from this, while protecting patients' privacy, might let me use many elements of psychoanalytic work that would otherwise remain unused, and might also enable my writing to bring together the theoretical and imaginative aspects in an entirely new form. This experience may make me feel freer from identification with one role – the analyst, the trainer, the person who is *writing* and is perhaps ambitious to be *a writer*, the assiduous and passionate reader, the person with her own history – and may allow me to slip to and from between them. I hope that without betraying any of these identities, I can reoccupy and respect them with their distinct "house rules," but without letting the rules stifle them, without shrinking the wide-open spaces that our priceless multiple and heterogeneous identities grant us and which the miracle of writing helps us understand and maintain over time as testimony of an experience sought and found.

In this way, Carine rises out of the writing as a character in her own right, but also as a patient *recognised* through writing and in the many other analytic experiences I have gone through on a daily basis. She is also a figure with whom I easily form countertransferential ties as I write about her, since her history is so redolent of my own.

Carine left Chile with her whole family shortly after the coup of 1973. She, her parents, and various uncles and aunts with their respective families moved to Italy, a country where her father had longstanding contacts as a naval engineer with a prominent role in the Chilean shipbuilding industry. His early sense of what was coming had enabled him to salvage enough of his property to reinvest it in a new profession which immediately became highly profitable. He was not equally adept at family life, where the enterprising one was Carine's mother, an artist with few prospects, born into wealth, a graduate in art history, and very religious like her sisters who had moved either to Italy or to California, which is where Carine would have preferred to go.

When she came to me asking for analysis, I was far from sure I was the right person or even that she needed an analysis, despite the insistence of all the dermatologists she had consulted that her problem was psychological. What strikes me at our first meeting, apart from the elegance and flimsiness of her dress, is her marked limp and highly disjointed posture. As soon as she sits down and takes off her dark glasses I see that the lenses were covering two big uneven scratches, one on each of her cheekbones. In a rather emphatic gesture, she puts the glasses on my table and says, "So here I am." I ignore the gesture and ask about "*her*" reasons for being there. She tells me she has been advised to come to me by a friend who is a doctor, and to whom she had confided that there was no dermatologist willing to pay serious attention to her acne, as she called it, and give her treatment for it. She had sudden pruritis *sine materia* all over her body with no organic reasons, despite repeated investigations, and it was making her scratch violently.

She gives me an "inverted gaze," a look I have identified in psychotic patients, but this time it takes me completely by surprise and leaves me a bit hesitant, as if I were the one oscillating between the meaning of words on the one hand and a facial expression on the other. She has sailed through her university career, gaining a first-class degree in medicine, and an indefatigable work ethic has carried her to the top of her profession which has been crowned with success. Her marriage ended badly but she has three wonderful children. In short, nothing accounts for that gaze into an internal abyss.

She asks me if I have any better medications than the ones she has been given by the dermatologists to control the effect of those lesions.

I say I'm afraid I must disappoint her: "I don't prescribe, but if you are interested, we can *treat them* together." And then in the silence I add, "The wounds are very painful," but she seems to deny this symbolic content. After another brief silence she starts to tell me about her arrival in Italy; her difficult start at school and the long absence the year after; the private Italian teacher who came to teach her at home while her mother refused to learn the language and went on speaking Spanish, mixing it with French as was her habit, as if change was impossible. At the end of the hour she struggles to stand up: her dress is flimsy and she seems almost to walk on tiptoe.

In the conversations that follow she keeps bringing up the question of the choice between dermatologists and the analyst. I point out to her that putting a dermatologist and an analyst together is like putting together two parts of herself that are antithetical: a prescriptive doctor and the opposite. She says, "Well, this could definitely help me: the lesions and their opposite." And I am very hesitant in the face of the intense systems of splitting and denial that are present and the unconscious aggressiveness that appears pervasive, though accompanied by a highly syncretic symbolism that is *perhaps* emerging from her words and, if so, may open the way to hope. Some months later she has two dreams, after which we pass on to a less veiled analytic work.

First dream:

She is in a hospital bathroom. The room is very large and there is no door between the bedroom and the bathroom. The only door is behind her, and behind the WC. The WC has no seat and she can feel the marble chill of the porcelain on her skin. She produces hard white faeces like bits of plaster and then, independently, the WC flushes and takes everything away. It is a very powerful whirlpool that is sucking her down too: she is terrified but then realises I am behind the door and, overcoming the embarrassment that she might feel in that position, is glad that I am able to pull her out of the vortex.

She continues almost without a pause. The dream "*petrified*" her[7] with its potent set of meanings; she is still incredulous, intuiting that something is moving in the analysis. I say nothing and she goes on. She says the faeces are hers, her lumps of plaster – she's expelled them at last!! – but they still have power over her: they drag her away; if it had not been for my fortunate arrival "behind" the door, the whirlpool would have sucked her down. I point out to her that the room has no dividing walls, like life with her mother who has access to all areas. She changes her tone and says seriously, "I didn't tell you that I was born with a dislocated hip. Not serious, and some surgeons in Chile had said it could be corrected without surgery. My mother wouldn't put up with me like that. The defect was stunting my growth and would leave me with a limp. She had me operated on. That had a disastrous effect on my whole body because I contracted an infection in the bones which deformed my body and turned me into a monster. The problem was that I couldn't walk any more. I went through endless operations and spent years almost completely encased in plaster, sarcophagi of plaster where I spent whole years of my adolescence. Then I was kept out of school (other people mustn't see me); only *she* was going to look after me. It was hell. My dream was about hoping to escape from hell. And you were guarding the door I could go through, but I'm not yet able to do it."

"What about the cold porcelain of the WC with no seat?" I ask.

"Oh yes, that's a bit of the pain and the hell. When they cut me out of the plaster that was around almost my whole body, I felt enormous pain because the bones were struggling to set, and along with the pain I was feeling the cold of those porcelain beds in the plaster room. I was thinking, 'I'm dead, I'm in the morgue.' I didn't want anyone to touch me! I yelled and scratched, and there was only one nurse, a man as delicate as an angel, who could calm my fury. I could cry with him, but my tears and sobbing made the pain worse. At least my mother wasn't there."

Analyst:You put me behind you. Maybe that's what you want.
Patient:You're right. Maybe that means the analysis is beginning.
A:[8] You want to expel it from your body, that poorly digested plaster that colours your faeces white, but you're afraid that one part of you, which you don't control, may let you fall into a whirlpool. The door is an opening, but it is also a limit that contains this urge. It gives a boundary to these unbounded spaces where everything can invade and intrude.
P: I can't know if you would have come to help because the anxiety woke me up. But I know that your presence reassured me at first.
A: Well, maybe that's because I don't come in.

The intrusion of absence

The dream refers to the intrusive aspects of absence. The mother is present in the intrusive violence of the decisions about Carine's body and the damage that they caused. Perhaps for this very reason, the mother remains profoundly absent.

The analyst seems to be missing too, but the hope is that this might be a transformative lack since, by staying outside, her non-entry could allow a boundary to be defined, a limit to access, and encourage the start of a restructuring. In the dream it is given a reassuring function.

And yet there is still the prevailing destructive urge to be attuned and identified with the internalisation of a mother who wants to suck life out: an inversion of the breastfeeding function. It seems that Carine could be describing the almost physical power, perceptible on a bodily level, of this sucking urge,[9] as if the injuries, beyond what she is able to represent at a verbal level of development, could have much earlier origins during a developmental phase that was still between the somatic and the psychic.

Other hypotheses run through my mind. Perhaps Carine only wants to indicate the deep impact and the humiliating effect, as well as the mutilation, of the trauma on the physical level.

Thinking about my final quip – "Well, maybe that's because I don't come in" – I wondered how far I might have been pursuing the paradoxical thought which I was formulating at that moment: that the patient also wanted to project and impose a *bad enough mother* onto me.[10] Indeed, a first thought was that she wanted to keep the mother outside, as she had kept her out of the plaster room where the mother would have wanted to come in and interfere. I had been disturbed by the story, so it is easy to imagine how relieved I felt at being "outside," which in the dream seemed to be a strongly differentiating element between the mother and me, but at the same time it could distance me defensively from the patient exactly as her mother had been distanced. This feeling of relief at being outside, clinging onto a lot of very helpful correlatives derived from theory, has been a recurrent sensation in my countertransference with severely traumatised patients.

The link to theory has often been my reading of Green where, clearly differentiating it from the "maternal disinvestment" which occurs in the *dead mother* complex (1993), he talks about a "necessary non-investment" to which the mother's gaze must fleetingly turn but which is still in tune with what Winnicott says about the *good enough mother* (1965). Green specifies, as Laplanche also did with reference to the analytic relationship, that *indifference* actually means "equivalent attention" to every element of psychic life; not rejection, not disregard.

I also thought hard about how well I might identify with a *bad enough* mother who aims to intrude without excess, one whom the patient should, but also could, keep out. I am choosing the expression *bad enough* to indicate a "negativity" without traumatic excesses which may in turn indicate a *potential object*, an object that on the one hand can keep the subject away from a sucking and annihilating vortex, and on the other may later lead to a transformative and more inclusive transference.

Another dream:

"I'm at the hairdresser's. My hairdresser is like a friend, I've been going to her for so long now, but in the dream she's blonde. She's carefully washing my hair, massaging it gently, and then she carefully takes each strand, dividing them with combs, and rolling them with the brush before drying them. This operation usually hurts. But in the dream I feel the firmness of her hand and it doesn't pull, so I calmly let her comb my hair. While I'm so relaxed I suddenly feel my heart pounding fast. In the mirror I see another head, but it's a head seen from behind, not the face, and it's someone else, someone who's nearly bald. A few skimpy white hairs stick out from between horrible wrinkles. The hairdresser sees my horror and stops, but she doesn't stop me. I don't know where I find the courage, but I clutch those skimpy hairs to turn the face towards me and look it in the eyes. As I turn it I see it's a monk's face. I can't describe the expression! It's indescribably ferocious. I don't think I've ever actually seen something so terrifying. It opens its toothless, sneering mouth as if it wants to devour me, it's drooling. I don't feel protected by the mirror and, as I'm wondering what it's *reflecting*, where that real image is that I'm seeing in the mirror, the thundering of my heart wakes me up. I was sweating and I spent the morning counting the hours until my session. Oh, I was forgetting. At one point the monk points his index finger, but it's arthritic and knotted and deformed, and I don't understand what it's pointing to. All I see is a fingernail and it looks like a claw."

Out of the mirror: the denied "reflection"

The image in the dream seems to refer to an impinging gaze at the *mirror stage*,[11] Lacan's representation of the inaugural encounter with the other, and so to the impossibility of the Ego mourning himself like an object, as Freud described in *Mourning and Melancholia* (1915a). The importance of being mirrored in the mother is rightly noted by Winnicott too, and the risk of being mirrored in the void is described by Marie-Claude Lambotte as *the Ego outside the frame*.[12]

Therefore the point being raised here about *reflecting-mirroring* refers to the reflection in the mirror, of which the concepts just noted represent the possible correlatives in theory of an intrusion in the moment of development: but they also speak symbolically about damage to the capacities for "reflection" and thus about a lasting harm (though its extent cannot be evaluated) to the capacity for thinking.[13]

While someone is delicately looking after her *head*, Carine is in the same position as the analyst, *behind*, where she can see, *reflect*, and cause to be reflected in the mirror of interiority the most uncomfortable, dubious, and awkward parts that belong to her.

Perhaps this is not the only thing in the new mirroring. Perhaps the mirror also refers to elements of the analytic climate that Carine is already able to utilise as a restructuring factor. The hypothesis is suggestive, even if what Lacan calls the "mirror stage" still seems to be compromised. In the "mirror stage" the structuring element of subjectivity is the other's gaze which makes the baby feel he is the subject of that gaze, on the condition that he give up gazing at himself (a symbolic and representational sign that *primary narcissism* has been overcome and the capacity to mourn been achieved).

With regard to the monk, I thought of monks and nuns as Servants of Mary, Mother of God, a not insignificant move in relation to someone who said she had known hell with a mother who demanded divine perfection…

I was overcome by a mournful silence.

Remembering, repeating, and not working through

I have reflected at length on how trauma bursts into analytic sessions, repeating itself with imperceptible variations. This repeated evocation of the trauma in the session has convinced me how, in sharing the traumatic aspects, the analyst also finds herself countertransferentially living through similar repetitions in and out of the session, characterised above all by repeated thoughts: although in this case – at least, so we hope – it is a return *in* thought. In other words, it is a reprise in search of new pathways, rather than a compulsion to repeat the contents. Nevertheless, this requires a specific reworking in the countertransference which I will address in the closing sections of this chapter. Repetitive activity is the only active part preserved by the Ego which has undergone the trauma, since the defence of repression has to a large extent failed at the start under an excessive stimulus, as Freud also emphasised in the second seduction theory.

As happens in the *vendetta*, repetition tends to function both as a disorganising and destructive element and as an active element for the preservation of the Ego, a sort of primal prioritising of the Ego's survival.

What does repetition do for psychic survival? This question has perennially been asked by humankind through the celebration of recurrences, the careful repetition of rites of passage, and through the repetition of human behaviours abundantly recorded in the wisdom of folk sayings (see Chapter III). The observation of nature also highlights its inexorable repetitions, terrifying humankind when this return introduces unforeseen variations, such as the tragic climatic changes we are now witnessing, paradoxically caused by human beings themselves. The fruitful repetition of every new birth is balanced by the inexorable repetitions of every living being's end, since living can only be living if it reaches a conclusion and at some point turns into dying.

It is into this twin track of life and death that repetition is inserted, at least from a psychoanalytic viewpoint, with the possibility of attaining a further meaning which does not completely resolve the question but nevertheless opens up new interpretative scenarios.

Incidentally, on the subject of survival, I suggest there is a biological experience related to neuronal plasticity,[14] to be used here in a metaphorical sense.

An aging or diseased neurone defies the logical expectation that it will move steadily towards death. On the contrary, the neurone sets survival mechanisms in motion, similar to those used during the early phases of development, restructuring its connections and optimising its demands for energy, a process which may considerably prolong its existence in difficult conditions and even enable it to return to normal functioning if the environmental conditions improve.

Cellular functioning and even structure seem to acquire new modalities in order to master the traumatic event and the resulting threat to life that the trauma brings with it.

My idea is to call the Ego's mastering of trauma in this way *possessing the trauma.*[15] The mastery is initially characterised by the illusion of not having undergone a trauma and then, during analytic work, it may lead to a better management of repetition in which tiny transformations are introduced step by step. (For example, "I am the monk" asserts possession of a threatening reality that is intrinsic to a subject, a threat of being flayed alive by a nail-claw, and is already perhaps the first spark of disillusionment about the real possibility of the Ego mastering the threatening intrapsychic impulses.)

It seems to be the setting up of a priority that the Ego unconsciously establishes to guarantee its survival – a priority that is as sudden as it is gradual – although it is not always in a position to control the simultaneous appearance of a sadistic drive. (See the *multiplicity of the afflux of excitations* also cited in the definition of trauma by Laplanche and Pontalis, 1967.) So the repetition would be set up with the purpose of reducing the Ego's own functions to a minimum, likewise remoulding its structure – as in the metaphor of the neuronal cell – with the aim of guaranteeing its survival.

The Ego's traumatic affirmation necessarily comes before its pleasure but it is an indispensable condition for a hypothecated idea of future well-being. Survival becomes a priority for living, but may nonetheless be organised as an endless deferral of living.

The death instinct of repetition is thus inexorably entwined with the impulse to life.

If this is plausible, what is the terrible condition of *impasse* for analytic treatment?

On the one hand, it is compulsion to repeat in analysis, with a re-actualisation of the trauma in the transference onto the analyst-object (transference only onto the object).

On the other hand, an arduous struggle to overcome the difficulty in using repression.

On the first point, I believe that if the analyst knows how necessary it is to re-actualise the trauma, he also knows how to avoid challenging it and defending himself against it. It is interesting to see André Green endorsing the Freudian concept of using the object in the compulsion to repeat: the object is not the instrument for reaching the goal of desire but the means by which discharge is effected. This is also because the excitation of the trauma predominates, obscuring and often suppressing the desire. At this point I need to be more specific about the way the compulsion to repeat is interpreted in trauma, to add clarity to what has been said so far, and even more so to what is going to be proposed along the way. I think it is obvious by now that I am not talking about the compulsion to repeat as the expression of a dominant death instinct. Nevertheless, I want to stress that this interpretation of repetition in trauma, which is always a re-actualisation, does not exactly fit into the distinction proposed by many authors, and expounded with exemplary clarity by Michel de M'Uzan – first in 1970 and with revisions in 2017, a year before his death.

In *Le même et l'identique* de M'Uzan distinguishes between a repetition of the *same*, which is subject to possibilities of variation in its repeating, and the reiteration of the *identical*, which is doomed to immutability.

With Green, de M'Uzan's analytic brother-in-arms, I have found myself thinking that even the re-actualisation of what appears identical – and which the term re-actualisation in this context reinforces – may allow minute variations, for all the reasons that appear in this book and which I sum up as *possessing the trauma*, such as the insistence on the object to represent it. In support of this hypothesis, though following a different theoretical path, I also suggest Nathalie

Zaltzman's powerful idea of the *anarchic instinct* (2015). Zaltzman does not see a parallelism between life and death instincts, but rather a chiasmus and an asymmetry, through which the anarchic instinct manifests itself to demolish the repetitiveness of the evil. From this viewpoint, *Thanatos* would express its vital function through the anarchic instinct which enables resistance to extreme situations where there is a totalitarian dispossession at work in the collective and in the individual. (I revisit the compulsion to repeat in the work of Fachinelli in n25 of this chapter.)

In these moments of repetition in clinical work we must hypothesise that there is a discontinuity in the transference similar to what happens in psychosis, though different in intensity and duration, and especially in its metapsychological significance. In other words, the transference is more enacted on the object, through repetition, than conveyed in words. In my view, the abandonment of the transference into word happens within the traumatic experience, more in favour of a fleeting sadistic dominance by the Superego than through absolute abuse by a totalising inner object, a product that is now split from its origin in the Superego, in competition with the object of the transference, as mostly occurs in psychosis and results in a sharp separation from reality. Green also wished to differentiate the transference onto the object from the transference onto words, and I will return to this point later.

An approach that is careful rather than naïve allows this crowd of repetitions to flow while we try to foster the gradual construction over time of embankments to contain them. In this approach the figure of the analyst is in a position we could call *parallel* to the traumatic repetition, a position which in the case of Carine is underlined in the first of the two dreams which pictures the analyst as being outside the door. That is, it depicts the analyst as being there without obstructing: enabling free action, which is also free discovery. This position parallel to the trauma will also recur by way of other features emerging in the analysis. The parallel position protects the analyst from sadistic attacks and yet allows the patient to feel both the analyst's presence and her state of neutrality, and sometimes her necessary inertia.

This means patient and analyst sharing a sort of *narcissistic curfew*.[16]

As we know, the Mediaeval term "curfew" indicated a law aimed at the control of fires. It required domestic fires, streetlights, and lanterns to be extinguished overnight. This was a way of trying to reduce the risk of conflagrations starting accidentally since they would have a greater chance of spreading by night and causing substantial damage. In more recent periods of history it has been extended during wartime, both to control nocturnal movements and as protection against attacks from the air.

Used metaphorically, the term curfew vividly represents the state of war-conflict in action (on both fronts, internal and external) as well as the defence that is necessary for shared survival and can bring analyst and patient together to survive long periods of time spent waiting. It is also an expression that takes into account the scaling-down of forces. An analyst who is too strong, too defended, is like a wall against which the patient's waves break and crash back ruinously onto him, as Green reminds us both in his study of *borderline states* (*On Private Madness*, 1986) and in *Le temps éclaté* (2000).[17]

It is a condition of sharing and not of reciprocity.

Last but by no means least, the curfew is always imposed by an authority – like the lockdowns imposed to contain the pandemic – and in psychoanalysis it is still metaphorical. Is it the analytic rule? The setting? Both? In any case, these are evocative elements of Oedipal submission to the Law.

Similarly, overcoming the difficulty/impossibility of using repression cannot be promoted by the analyst adopting an active, directive stance. Patients who come into analysis are usually endowed with sufficient capacity for libidinal investment but, as always, this is not generalisable, especially now that the clinical typology has been extended to situations which place the analytic couple in ever greater *difficulty* (and I want to stress the choice of this term as opposed to the more commonly used *severity*, which is both generic and customarily applied only to the Other, the patient). And as I see it, this can make a difference to the likelihood of overcoming the trauma. Highlighting a latent or dormant or narcissistically abandoned investment, session after session, and especially in dreams, is not an easy thing to do. And yet this is the way to *weave a fabric in parallel to the trauma* which may make it possible to draw on a world of phantasies that brings subjectivating resources and permit a movement beyond survival, not leaving the subject in the stalemate of deferred living that can become endless. As time passes, the composing of these features may itself function as a container of repetition and traumatic re-actualisation, and in this way the containing feature will also have a structural function, setting a limit, an alternative boundary.[18] But all this may only take shape as a far-off destination.

The starting point can be a large, murky, inexorable swamp because of a repetition that is hard to circumvent since its boundaries are constantly blurred in the psychic mist.

We can assume that Carine had a childhood and adolescence marked by her mother's obsessions about the menace of contaminations from public swimming pools, prohibitions against her daughter using the toilets at school, and a series of other restrictions and constant, torturing controls. All this led to serious consequences for Carine's excretory functions, and inevitably also for her sexual development, her sexuality, and her social relationships, having been alone and isolated since she was very young.

Repetition in her sessions was characterised by years of prolonged silence, an active silence, sometimes a very long pause in her thinking, a void made of accumulated indigestible material, like the severity of her constipation in childhood, but also a traumatic excess that emptied her of the ability to let herself go, to make her body and speech flow, which could only be put back in motion once many years of analysis had reset her biological and psychic clocks into synchrony.

When the analysis is quite far advanced she brings another dream which bears wonderfully vivid witness in pictographic and figurative form to the theoretical path that has sustained the analytic couple.

She is involved in an investigation about a catastrophic event. There has been a flood. A mudslide has submerged and destroyed an entire town but people have been able to flee in time. There are many survivors wandering around the muddy remains. She wants to write a denunciation of the irresponsible *Institutions*, which she associates with her parents, but she is dissuaded by Hans who tells her that this is the moment for solidarity and reconstruction. (Hans was a Jewish next-door neighbour from her childhood, a survivor of the Nazi extermination who fled to Marseilles alone as a young child and then made his way to Latin America. He has already on several occasions been interpreted in analysis as a father with auxiliary functions.) Carine glimpses me in the distance and this reassures her. She says "in the distance" and then immediately specifies that I am "in the rear." She notes that when I change position I move in two different ways, but always keeping a discreet distance and staying in the rear: sometimes parallel to the flow of the mud, sometimes at a right angle to it, and incisive in the instructions I am giving to the civil authorities.

We are both struck by the transferential-countertransferential weight of this dream and it puts energy into a benign movement that will stay with us to the end.

Even today, years later, I am still struck by the strategic-theoretical intensity of this dream, a strategy that can only be re-read *après-coup*. I have been thinking about how Carine's unconscious, in the very long, very distressing moments of silence, had been able to record, memorise, and keep hold of her and my psychic movements as mnemic traces in the uproar of those silences, the uproar of war, audible and unmistakable even in the rearguard. The rearguard covers the army at the back, and behind Carine there always loomed a menacing and enduring sadistic Superego that had held together a fragile, hobbling Ego, and she had surrendered to it for years. But in the vanguard there was the subject who, after the traumatic experience of feeling deprived of any subjectivity, resulting in self-doubt on all fronts from the sexual to the professional to the social, had fought the battle to regain her subjectivity with the help of an existential guide.

Like Liliana Segre[19] who, finding herself in a position to kill her enemy, gives up her revenge and chooses life, so Carine listens to Hans and sets off to rebuild her life.

The long, slow parallel movement corresponds to the need to repeat the trauma in sessions: time passes in parallel to the flow of mud, does not obstruct it, and is not disrupted by it. Neither the subject nor the transference-object is immersed in the mudslide: they are present, always visible, can always be kept in view. The analyst shares the drama of the trauma but does not put herself in the midst of the mudflow, and this becomes a suggestion that the patient can keep herself out of it. In any case, the analyst never abandons her post, and follows the flow.

Among the many meanings of the term *compassion*[20] identified by Antonio Prete in his literary and poetic revisiting of it, to which I refer the reader, I would add that it is not only *being close to pain* (Latin: *patior*, Greek: πάθος) but also closeness to and sharing of transitions and steps; and also bringing-into-being through sharing (like the curfew in the session) the possibility of passing beyond (Hebrew: פסח, *pesach*, *pâsâchti*).[21] However, in these parallel passings, close but parallel, there would be no opening to the new (Latin: *pateo*) without the incisiveness of a word that is perpendicular to the trauma and penetrates from outside, prompting the mudflow onto a different course, fostering a "civil" organisation of the bodily functions and "civil" protection, thereby fostering an acceptable coexistence of mind and body.

In the chapter of his book *Compassione* (2013) entitled "Metamorphosis," Antonio Prete writes,

> So, for poetry, its principal language – that is, metaphor – is profoundly concerned with metamorphosis. The multiform nature of possible change, Valéry called it in a passage from his *Cahiers*. The loss of the ego, of shape, and of language that is displayed in metamorphosis rocks the imagination: the sympathy for this transition and the disturbance caused by the void that accompanies any slippage of form testify to the way that, whenever this happens, it calls into question the self's belonging to itself, the defined corporeality of one's own senses, and the perception of singularity, of being unrepeatable.[22]
>
> (pp. 79–80)

Antonio Prete follows direct and oblique trajectories of compassion, as is mentioned on the back cover of his book, and the author himself describes a humanisation which we could call horizontal and "a representation of compassion that is, so to speak, vertical" (ibidem., 12) to underline this intricate, changeable, and controversial advance along a path that passes through human pain and its transformation.

But would all this have been possible if the analyst had not used a *lateral transference*? – i.e., Hans, an auxiliary figure in the patient's transference but complementary to the work of the analyst's countertransference.

I think that in difficult situations which almost always accompany gross traumas, or events experienced as annihilating attacks which imprison the subject in a repetition with no way out, attention to what reality brings in the form of the representable and complementary is the only way out of the real – understood as concrete, unsymbolisable, and unrepresented – that gets wedged into the psyche like a peg that blocks the development of thinking.

Theoretical, clinical, and methodological reflections

Before we can attain these good possibilities for development which, speaking in a spirit of disillusionment, I know are very fortunate outcomes since the opposite can easily be the case, the representation that is set up by unfruitful circumstances may for a long time remain in the analytic relationship, and in the analyst, as a threat. In the early phases of the process an immense place is represented in the analyst's mind, almost an infinite desert where every horizon is merged with all the others, a long, boundless plain devoid of trees and with no hills to vary the eyeline, an eternity of standing in a foggy marshland where the swampy surface is treacherous and the mist obscures every possible way out. The scenario in my mind which I have tried to describe is very like that of Andrei Tarkovsky's film *Stalker*.[23] The director had been in voluntary exile from the USSR since 1970 but had asked to go back so he could make this film in a prohibited area. In the film the area is prohibited because an asteroid had landed there, but it was actually a zone contaminated by radiation, a fact that was not without consequences for the company. The marshy terrain and endless mist are characteristic of the setting in which the film was made. An anxious, almost incessant sense of lost boundaries dominates the viewer's experience.

In analytic work too, the threat is not represented but enacted by means of an image that remains mute. Sometimes, however, speech "presents" itself with a word enacted in the gap which André Green called the *halo of speech*, hence a transitional zone to and from the thing, but also a transit towards a possible representation of that still silent nucleus.

I have tried to record the mutterings perceived in the session, perhaps the hint of smiles, as equivalents of possible access to free associations that are achieved later, and as Freud suggests in *Analysis Terminable and Interminable* (1937a), as a first moment of contact with the patient and their internal movement.

The *narcissistic curfew* is thus a stable position, but neither inert nor without points of reference: it stays parallel to the possibility of using all the cognitive baggage while the active-repetitive part of the trauma is still present with the usual traumatic repetitions and the old defences.

Possessing the trauma is the first defence of the patient's Ego, the affirmation of the Ego that is trying to resist and survive being cut loose by the death instinct which continues to foster the irruption of a traumatic excess into the psyche, an irruption whose pervasive affective charge, free and overflowing – cut loose, indeed – cannot be linked to representation, cannot gain access to the symbolic: and at the same time, and for the same reasons, it cannot be repressed. Despite this, the Ego does not surrender to the failure of all these psychic possibilities, but hypothecates them by insisting on the object without yet being able to represent it. In *Inhibitions, Symptoms and Anxiety* (1926), Freud, now seventy and suffering recurrent attacks of angina pectoris, thinks back to Ernst and emphasises that the boy learns to differentiate powerlessness in the face of danger – *Hilflosigkeit* – from the possibility of mastering the danger by anticipating it. Freud differentiates a real danger that is foreseeable from the instinctual danger that is less foreseeable.

This repeated alternation which, as Green reminds us, is never identical to the previous repetition, represents an effective mobilisation of the Ego, even in the compulsion to repeat, through an unconscious attempt to latch on to the object, insisting on it, to recover some mnemic traces that may allow a future reconnection to the symbolic and the representable for the purposes of phantasmatic investment.

In my view, the symptom, like play, has a fundamental capacity for redeeming the Ego which has suffered the excitation that follows trauma. The passivity of not being able to effect a change to the crushing and distressing experience has in fact mobilised an activating internal excitation on both the purely somatic-instinctual and psychic levels which, in non-traumatic conditions, is devolved to investment in a phantasmatic representation.

But it can take a very long time to evolve in this direction.

The theoretical image of *possessing the trauma*, in its passing from the somatic-instinctual to a possible representation in phantasy, can be set alongside Bollas's concept of *the unthought known*,[24] a condition intrinsic to the body Ego of the early developmental stages in which the mother becomes the transformative object: that is, she introduces and induces a process in the Ego so that it gradually acquires structure and makes her an object. Bollas is thinking about a form of knowledge founded chiefly on sensory and affective elements which are expressed as a bodily *idiom*, which becomes active in adult life, being associated and interwoven with the cognitive processes more properly belonging to the secondary process, but also capable of reappearing separately from it.

The theoretical hypothesis which I propose for the analytic process encounters some moments that I would call transitional in terms of thinking – touching on both Freud's *primary narcissism* and Bion's *rêverie*, though they are recalled here with respect for their specific character, and they remain specific theoretical concepts in their own right[25] – to support an Ego which, if it is to survive a traumatic attack, must deploy all its energies of counterinvestment: and, as I mentioned earlier, in such a mobilisation of the instincts the sadistic instincts may find the way open to them for combining to pervert the goal.

We must also take into account the fact that the repetitions are centred on a traumatic plurality, of which only the tip of the iceberg is visible. Some traces remain submerged and will only appear much further into the analytic process. The traces will also remain entirely silent because they refer to previous traumas whose existence may be postulated through the patients' description of the absence or inadequacy of maternal care, or through the characteristics of certain symptoms: digging into the skin, for example, which symbolises both an intrusive penetration from even earlier in life and a desire to dig for freedom, while at the same time being an indelible trace on the body, a bodily idiom, a script in the body. These traces can also be associated with disturbances of the primary bodily functions that persist in adulthood or with certain disturbances of the identity. Kris[26] holds that the earlier the traumatic experiences and the more archaic the material which appears in the analytic process, the more widely its derivatives manifest themselves across a range of behaviours, and in these patients they are indeed multiple. He also maintains that the broader the base on which the analysis can build a specific reconstruction of early experiences and archaic impulses – in other words, the more fruitful the analytic work – the greater the probability of awakening their global effect in the session. This risk, as in everything I have said so far, relates to the inevitable condition of partial passivity in the analyst and in the analytic couple; a passivity which, though partial, cannot be ignored.

(I am referring to the complex concept of passivity proposed by Levinas and to how the analytic couple is consequently exposed to a vulnerability. These are theoretical positions which I feel add weight to my idea of the *narcissistic curfew* in sessions during the re-actualisation of the trauma.)

So, *possessing the trauma* is a theoretical image as much concerned with the Ego's attempt to counter-invest the traumatic aggression and guarantee its own survival – albeit with a life hypothecated into the future – as with the analyst's difficult operation of integrating two functions: standing at the edge of the traumatic abyss without plunging into it by re-actualising the traumatic repetition, and attempting an autobiographical reconstruction which has not yet found a suitable expressive possibility and a sublimatory investment to describe it.[27]

Even so, what inner journeys has the analyst made in her countertransference work to make possible this *position parallel to the trauma?*

What defences are being mobilised in the analyst? How does she work on them? How do they encounter those of the patient?

The theoretical image of *narcissistic curfew* tries to describe all this, not so much by replying to these questions as by looking for theoretical and methodological instruments that may ensure they are always bearable, capable of being addressed, and helpful in considering psychoanalysis as a therapeutic garrison which, though it is not the only one, is nevertheless indispensable in traumatic situations. The curfew is an image that seeks to integrate the various aspects of temporality in therapeutic care while also bringing a sense of care to that *impasse* which traumatic experience insists on.

Several authors have addressed this *impasse.*

Though the drive theory is a foundation stone of this study, it has also been inevitable that I should think about other authors who have asked themselves the question, more or less explicitly, about how to pass through the repetitive *impasse* and how to position oneself while waiting and looking for a way out. So I have been accompanied in these reflections at different times by Winnicott, Bion, Bromberg, Roussillon,[28] Aulagnier, and others. This is not because I have a taste for hybridisation but rather because of the idea, which I endorse, of a necessary cooperation between theories, even though it inevitably involves conflict, as I have already suggested in Chapter I.

In this connection, I often find myself suggesting the architectural metaphor of the vaulted arch, an arch in which the lines converge on a single point, the strongest point of the whole structure, but stability is given by the fact that these lines rest on points that are distinct, opposed. It is the same for theories which in general cannot converge but can support each other, meeting each other at certain points while also remaining distinct and separate.

This is what I mean when I try to define *theoretical complementarity.*

The aim of theoretical-clinical writing, but I would say of any psychoanalytic text, is to expose oneself to comparison and verification, as Green often reminds us. Every analytic experience needs theory if it is to be translated into working instruments which can be shared and compared with others, instruments that are open to criticism and confutation, key elements of any scientific procedure.

I had Ernst's game in mind, and Freud's reflections on it, and I thought about using it not as a way of anchoring myself faithfully to the past, but as a *theoretical roof.* In his repetition of the cotton-reel game, Ernst tries to bind the anti-entropic energy of the death instinct and, in doing so, makes the lack of the object tolerable while also putting its rediscovery into play. In this sense, I felt I was a granddaughter, daughter of another generation, separated from the father, although linked to the origins of his thought. So I had in mind a *theoretical roof* under which the *narcissistic curfew* is situated like a sort of virtual *cloud*, a large container understood, as Roussillon suggests, as a transformative envelope where one can deposit the material that is discharged without having been worked through.

With these patients, in the silence of my own thoughts, I often found myself using the expression, "Let's hold it there," which referred to the countless repetitions enacted on the transference-object more than onto the word, but which also extended to all the phantasies and theoretical reflections that had a supportive function for me in the most difficult moments and nourished the epistemophilic impulse of sublimation, an element of pleasure which compensated me for the long wait and the disruptive elements of the repetition. I would call it *remaining* rather than *resisting*, and in this respect too my attachment to little Ernst emphasises his remaining in the traumatic situation of separation. I choose *remain* for its Indo-European root in the verb "MAN" which means "to think": in other words, to remain in analytic thinking.[29]

And *remaining* is neither to be taken for granted nor easy to do.

Other authors have wondered how to *remain* in traumatic repetition and, as I have already recalled, they have accompanied me on my reflections.

For Bion[30] it is the analyst's mind that takes on and expresses the capacity for becoming the container of the material which has not been worked through by the patient and, at the same time, expresses the capacity for remaining open to new possibilities: containing, but at the same time fostering, the processes of integration and the links of knowledge. Overall, it is the capacity for repression on the patient's behalf when the patient's contact barrier is deficient.

For Bromberg[31] the position is somewhat different. The analyst must defend himself, otherwise he will not survive the attacks of the traumatic repetitions: but he must also know that by doing this he may activate a degree of retaliation. Bromberg sees the working-through of an early trauma as fundamentally relational and it does not free the patient from what was done in the past, but from *what someone has to do to live with* what has happened in the past (*The Shadow of the Tsunami*, 2011).

Roussillon[32] also poses the problem of the analyst's survival in what he more generically terms "the so-called negative transference" (to which I will return) and says simply that analysts must free themselves from the transference, both negative and positive, in order to preserve a degree of creativity and hence of vitality.

I will start from this position to define my own which is both close to and detached from all three.

As I have maintained, the repetition that evokes the traumatic event, which is not necessarily the repetition of the traumatic event in itself, is inevitable; and, as I have tried to maintain, it is also necessary since it is the residue of an active part that the Ego has preserved in the traumatic experience, within the passivity of the trauma that has been undergone. This active part (*possessing the trauma*), which hypothecates into the future the possibility of working through and reorganising the traumatic event, is also a victim of this illusion since the compulsion to repeat is not a real move forwards but a discharge which can never fully set aside the traumatic perception, and so the subject is compelled to relive it, at least partly. The subject cannot then find a place for representation of the traumatic event, which would instead be a transformed psychic reiteration, and this deformation-transformation would use up a large quantity of the affect that might otherwise be free, thereby blocking the necessary disorganising effect.

Thus there is still no space where the internal perception can look for mnemic traces and where these traces can be reworked in phantasy so that the subject is once again central to this construction and opens up access to the symbolic, as Laplanche and Pontalis remind us.

One central question is posed in the *narcissistic curfew*, encouraged by the reflections of the authors named earlier: how to live the analytic experience and keep it alive during the compulsion to repeat. For a long time the object, and in particular the transference-object that is the analyst, is not a goal but an instrument of the repetitive discharge, and so the transference is not kept intact either onto the object or onto speech/the word, but is modified into what I would call a *discontinuous transference*.

I go back to Roussillon's claim that analysts must free themselves from both the positive and the negative transference. He does not mean we can work without transference; rather, I believe he is indicating the need to free oneself from an excessive concentration on the transference at the risk of objectifying it, losing its dynamicity, and, as in the case of repetitive traumatic acts, also losing the complexity and difficulty experienced in this *discontinuity from speech*. Roussillon critiques the definition of *negative transference*, and I feel the need to endorse this critique by proposing the *discontinuous transference* since it is not that the transference is diminished or turns negative, but if by *positive transference* we mean a transference that is always onto both the object and onto the word, in these critical situations there is a loss of such integration, from which this disconnection derives, a more or less substantial and more or less enduring discontinuity. Indeed, in these cases, the word is not representational but remains concrete, repeated and enacted in repetition like any other action.

So the question cannot be whether or not to free oneself from the negative transference, incurring the risk of possible retaliation against the patient, but neither can it mean thinking of oneself as a container without limits by maintaining a constant openness and unsaturability.

Thus, my proposed *narcissistic curfew* means hypothesising, under the umbrella of theory, an additional space for storing unelaborated repetitive material, a virtual cloud that may be drawn upon when a later return of mnemic traces makes phantasy and representation possible, and with them the temporality-atemporality of the unconscious. It is also the way to think about a possibility of remaining in analytic treatment, preserving a space for the pleasure of thinking, thanks to the mind's *thirdness* function.

Although these patients seem rich in artistic and cultural interests, it also seems that they can never fully enjoy them: that is, their interests seem to stand *in place of real libidinal investments* as if they were stereotypes to be offered to a social reality so that it could accept them in this embellished form, and make them welcome.

Instead, even after a prolonged experience of analysis, they seem to vibrate deeply with certain affects and I have sometimes had the impression that much of this may remain submerged as an inexpressible desire and that phantasy about it is still impossible.

First steps

As the analytic process unfolds Carine has a dream:

Her aunt, who has now been dead for years, was standing behind her and, with a very delicate, almost imperceptible gesture, was holding onto her, supporting her by the arms.

Carine associates the image in the dream with a childhood photo she had recently rediscovered. In the photo she is a toddler taking her first steps and her aunt is supporting her delicately, almost invisibly, from behind. A modification of the transference seems to be being sketched out, indicating the time it has taken "to make the first steps" and the analyst's inevitable, even if transitory, "supporting" function (equally inevitable is the link to Winnicott's *holding*), a support limited to presence, listening, and thinking. The aunt was a constant point of reference while she was alive and supported Carine in her many amorous misadventures whereas her mother used to denigrate her, considering her responsible for what was happening to her and saying she was always unworthy of the romantic relationships she embarked on. Carine was in fact possessed by the constant need to challenge her mother. She knew she was burdened by an inexorable judgement of herself as wretched, worthless, guilty of deformity, and without dignity; and all she could see was the need to battle "blindly" against this: blindly being the operative word, and we will soon see why.

In fact, and against her will, Carine had taken on many of her mother's characteristics, identifying unconsciously with her, perhaps to control her own destructive potential. The forms of functioning that were apparently the opposite of her mother's, and mostly based on reaction formations, seemed to have enabled an opposition on the part of her Ego: more through the confluence and precipitation of sadistic impulses in the service of a tyrannical and punitive Superego than through integrative and constructive movements in favour of real independence. None of these seemed to have given her much room for sublimation and transformation in support of a pleasure free from persecutory "games." Even her libidinal investment in her job had been badly polluted by the competitive need to assert herself and, because of her abilities, she had not run into major obstacles that might prompt criticism of her. Indeed, Carine's frustrations in this sphere were extremely rare. She had instantly achieved prestigious positions and was universally esteemed and admired.

She discovers *writing*, and only tells me about it after several years of analysis. She had started writing something that was not exactly a diary but rather her own story repeated endlessly, always with new variations, in coloured notebooks which she changed annually, and every book had to contain *everything*, "the whole story." As she said herself, most of the variations were fantastical, but real episodes and reflections on them were associated with these: i.e., mirror images of an inner reality in eternal flight from outward reality. The details changed, but there was always a rigorous subdivision into chapters: childhood, adolescence, university, marriage. Or else the chapters were arranged by subject: mother, aunt, husband, etc. For a long time this was how the sessions went, in chapters, as if representing a structural defensive tendency to categorise, to catalogue, to impose extreme order on something that corresponded to a tumultuous obstruction and a disruptive urge to disorganisation and disorder.[33]

In quite an advanced phase of her analytic journey it will be possible for Carine to work out that she was writing to testify; but before that it was just a way to take account of and assert her being-there, to affirm and firm up an identity in transition, one that was subjected to continual oscillations which made her feel she was merely "passing through," since she was unable to link "facts" to an identity of her own or to something more intimate that might belong to her.

She also wrote to make herself visible through writing in a sort of freeze-frame image, and as a way to make a tragic cross-section of this "passing through" emerge in the story.

I shall confine myself here to analysing the dual role of this writing, which is in fact something many patients do in parallel to their analysis. In my view it can unite the search for recognition and the affirmation of a history, the patient's history, with a sublimatory function which is not yet able to make any headway and often ends up lapsing into repetition. The patients' stories, which have been the only way I can get to know the characteristics of such writing, are therefore impregnated with the patients' judgements on their own evolution.

The discovery of these pages which describe hidden parts of Carine is in fact a rediscovery and revisitation taking place several years after they were written, and Carine now knows how to read and remember them in an entirely new spirit.

Out of the story there seems to emerge a willingness to construct a new sublimated version of the trauma, as well as a willingness to bear witness to her failure and the inexorable relapse into endless rewriting. In other words, there seems to be a prevailing illusion of preserving a memory that, on the contrary, is regularly lost since it is not a matter of recollections but of re-actualisations which, outside of analysis, do not find their transformative path.

Only towards the end of the analysis will Carine be able to comment that in the first years of analysis it was as if she had written a treatise, with a full commitment to reorganising things, in a sort of simultaneous unveiling and concealment.

So she was confronting two parts of herself, present in a highly unsettling duality. In fact, Carine was revealing a vertiginous distance between the writing being scarified on her body by dermographism – a symptom which had come to a definite end after the first two years of analysis – and the writing on paper. She was identifying a temporality suspended between the two parts of her, as if there were a profound difficulty with integration. Then the repeated flights of thought pondered in analysis seemed to fill this deep temporal gap, and the abyssal features of the gap between these differences were absolutely evocative of the traumatic element which characterised them.

In these patients the trauma sustains the abyss, but it is also at the base of the two functionings: the traumatic repetition and re-actualisation, and the attempt at autobiographical reconstruction supported by a libidinal-sublimatory investment which, for a long time, finds no adequate path to expression.

Psychic temporality

I will now set out a further reflection on the concept of temporality. The question of temporality has infused the history of psychoanalysis ever since the writings of Freud. Freud clearly demonstrated the centrality of the temporal in psychoanalysis, beginning with the fundamental rule and the fact that when movement starts to happen in the psyche, it is based on the overturning of differentiations between different kinds of time. In addition, he emphasised its extreme complexity.

In the two models, and especially in developing the three psychic agencies, Freud did not abandon the Kantian spatiotemporal system, but he did throw it into crisis with the unconscious atemporality expressed in dreams and neurosis; and also, we can surely add, in every symptomatic manifestation.

If we follow post-Freudian thought (for example, Gilles Deleuze in *Différence et répétition*, 1968) it leads the reader to think about a temporality registered originally in the body as part of instinctual life – the life and death instincts: a primitive temporality, a "blind" time reduced to one pulse and remote from the modulations of temporal consciousness. However, the Freudian oeuvre contains no unified treatment of spatialised time, continuous time, time in continuity with consciousness, and discontinuous time – the unconscious's time outside time – so this further investigation is left to his successors.

The theme of trauma adds a character of excess, unpredictability, and immediacy to this temporal complexity, as Freud himself stresses in his 1914 definition, with an effect that pierces the psychic structure; an effect that damages temporality itself, reducing it to an endlessly identical repetition, an endlessly current constant with no history.

The lacerating attacks brought by the trauma against the psyche cause the systems of repression to fail, and likewise all the temporal revisitings that occur with the return of the repressed and as a result of which the secondary processes preserve the ability to remodel the material which emerges.

Following the trauma, infantile amnesia will not be overcome as a whole, which we find Freud admitting with evident disappointment in 1937. Hence the hypothesis that what it has not been possible to repress, and thus locate in the potential to return in the form of recollections – because the material precedes the verbal phase – returns in the form of hallucinatory reminiscences, a sort of *decodification with no translation*: or as I would rather imagine it, a form of *transliteration* of the early traumatic phenomena (cf. the untranslatable remainder proposed by Laplanche).

Going back to Freud once again, he maintains that the analytic method is a psychic method but that symptoms, however much they may dominate, are not only psychic but also somatic: we could say that the two levels are inextricably mingled.

For his part, Green claims it is difficult to escape the impression that in the compulsion to repeat there is a regression to the most primitive stages of instinctual functioning, those that are closest to the return to the undifferentiated state and to its biological underpinning. It must follow from this, however, that the Freudian conception of time implies an integration on several levels of functioning: from the Id to the Superego, from primary to secondary to tertiary, in continual interaction with a biological element and its becoming psychic.

The various theoretical developments in Freud's thought thus distance themselves from the linearity of time in consciousness, which he sees as characterised by unidirectionality and the inexorable progression towards old age and death. Through the association of biological and psychic determinants, a *polychrony* comes to be composed before the reader's eyes, the expression of a multifariously extended temporality.

So this was Freud's revolutionary intuition: to bring to light the psyche's totipotency, which can thus resist the deterioration of its processes by time. In this way the psyche can suppress the disillusioning effects caused by the passing of real life and compensate its desires through dreams, phantasies, and the sublimating totipotency of thoughts.

Even so, it is impossible to offer a psychoanalytic theory of time without acknowledging a *time of the other*, and in *Le Temps éclaté* (2000), using a range of instruments, Green fills in some theoretical features missing from Freud's thought. The first experiences of time which arise for the pleasure principle are rooted in temporal sequences punctuated by rhythms and pauses.[34] If we consider the *time of the other*, what emerges is the other's potential for giving meaning, for offering a temporal arrangement and making it available through a succession of pleasant and unpleasant experiences, as well as doing the opposite: traumatically disorganising the structuring of temporality in the still-forming subject. According to Green, this all requires us to revisit the conception of time and it offers the possibility of a new look at every previous diagnostic classification. This revisiting of the varied temporal organisations that characterise the main groups of psychic functioning – normality, neurosis, borderline states, and psychosis – provides another valuable theoretical resource with a clinical consequence: that of leading us inevitably to a synchronous gaze, since all the mechanisms of temporal functioning in any psychic structure may be simultaneous, synchronous, and conflictual at the same time, while also being diachronous. What I would like to emphasise most strongly, because of its relation to trauma in clinical work, is the difference between atemporality and the denial of time which is so well-represented in the compulsion to repeat.

All the activities of the body and the psyche are obliged to acknowledge their decline, but the activity of the unconscious's atemporal function consists in the possibility, never lost and always potentially active, of reinvesting them. Desires and phantasies are part of our unconscious and, as Green also reminds us, are something that never gets used up, a constant reservoir of life and hope. This precise and complex psychic organisation, which enables desire to be articulated in phantasy in the atemporality of the unconscious, links still unfulfilled desires to the waiting that has already been accomplished, so as to have recourse to them in life's difficulties.

Does this mean, therefore, that the compulsion to repeat can enter into a form of atemporality?

Thanks also to the thinking of Green, I am convinced that the opposite is the case. The compulsion to repeat is not mere ignorance of time, or the refusal to admit its limitations, nor is it simply an omnipotent rebellion against it: instead it represents an arrest of time's forward march; we could call it a *murdering of time*. The destruction of hated objects also destroys the temporal processes connected to them, but at the same time paradoxically wants to stop the death of the object. To this end, Green has come up with the idea that the way to satisfy these contradictory demands is to freeze the experience of time and negate the phantasies connected to it. Finding an object, as Freud point out, means *re*-finding it, which implies having seen it before and an inevitable measuring of time.

It is precisely this dogged preservation of the object, the sole condition for the Ego's survival in trauma, that I use as the basis for my hypothesis of repetition's dual valence, and how this can simultaneously both damage the Ego and be an indispensable condition for saving it, recovering the object, and thus caring for it.

Carine has a dream which marks one of these transitions.

"I go out of the Hospital and head for the end of the street. It is a lovely Spring day and from the high wall of the Botanical Garden

I can see reeds and rushes waving, and I smell a scent of stock; at the end of the street I come to Piazza dei Miracoli, and I feel a real miracle working inside me: I'm healed! The piazza is wonderful."

Rushes are not native to Tuscany but, along with cacti and other succulents, they are originally from other continents. Stock, however, is Mediterranean: it grows near the sea and carries on its leathery stem the scars of leaves it has previously lost. It prefers chalky places and readily grows even on cliffs at the sea's edge or along walls, making do with very little earth. I decide not to interpret this and, to moderate the emphatic tone, I just comment on "the analysis of miracles" to remind Carine what analysis "never is."

The transference object is still idealised and the re-finding of a narcissistic Ego-object clearly shows how damaged it was and that it is still full of scars. Before moving on, there is a need to stay in the "negative." In fact, what is becoming operative here is the first attempt at *flight*: "I'm healed" seems to mean "I don't need analysis anymore," like her past urges to flight which have always been wholly irrational and, under the seeming cover of survival, have put the Ego in harm's way: "At last I can live and manage on my own." These were illusions of autonomy while adequate defences were still missing.

However, I have always detected a strong mixture of instincts in these impulses, which made me understand how indispensable they were for survival: the survival of a subjectivity which could only be revealed in this way.

I confined myself to "being there."

So flight was the cut-off, the always dramatic conclusion, the break, and above all the sign of activity being asserted over the experience of passivity: it was both the trace of the mother's psychosis and simultaneously the flight from it and opposition to it. Flight was the trauma of closeness to the maternal psychosis, borne by an individual who, "given birth by her and living close to her," finds herself experiencing it from early childhood without the defences she needed to deal with it.

So it was this necessary transgression which, in the transference, took the form of the long flight from free associations. The working-through of the flight was repeatedly attempted for a long time but this insistent need, this *possessing the trauma*, which she had probably kept alive through letting herself be crushed by the will of others, always seemed to be a matter of survival at all costs and at the same time evidence of a transferential dynamic: "I am in flight, but behind me there is someone waiting for me." This was all fully visible but, for a huge period of time, visibility was not enough for her to work out how to change.

Certainly the elements of the compulsion to repeat, as parts of a temporality which kills living time and makes the atemporality of *fantasieren* and phantasying unusable, were vividly apparent to me in this analysis and in other situations of massive early trauma. During the long phases of *narcissistic curfew* I had probably more than once put myself in tune[35] with these flights: flights from reality, flights from the commitments suggested by reality, and, above all, flights from the historical temporality of reality which imposes deadlines, verification times, conclusions of projects, new openings. In these long moments everything seemed to stop so that it could live somewhere else: a somewhere else that did not justify itself as an understandable flight from something feared and fearful, but was proposed-imposed as a triumph, as a way to celebrate a liberation, though it was more often evidence of the opposite.

In my experience of analytic work I do not in fact recall any true satisfaction from triumphs of this kind: the real rejoicings at freedom from pathological functioning have almost always been accompanied by sorrow over losses left unmourned. Lastly – and this last thing is not really last – while still in the *narcissistic curfew* I had interrogated my countertransferential work in the discontinuity of the transference. How far, I wondered, were my thinking and writing about these patients also an expression of my flight from them, my defence, my subterranean flight to the same curfew that sometimes made the stalemate unbearable to me? Instead of staying in a position parallel to the trauma, how often was I fleeing into a divergent, narcissistic position, sustained more by a reaction formation of my own than by completed sublimatory investment?

However, in the light of having worked through these clinical events I believe that between what I experienced in the session and what I was able to work through there is a gap that evades investigation, a level of darkness, not only in terms of answers but also of questions.

There have been other moments that were similar to flight but differed in being passed through by means of words.

Another of Carine's dreams:

The patient finds herself in a museum containing lots of stone statues that show the way to the picture gallery. She finally reaches the room that contains the paintings, and the passage that leads into it is marked by a glass corridor through which delightful frescoes and Gobelin tapestries can be seen on the walls, but no framed pictures. At the end of the corridor, which is L-shaped, she sees her own portrait hanging on the glass.

But it's more than that: it's a bust; the arms and hips are visible but not the legs. She feels intense astonishment but also anxiety and unease which do not wake her up, however.

In the associations she recalls that, among the statues leading to the entrance, there is one of *Cupid and Psyche*. Her comment on the glass gallery is about the transparency of her life, overcoming the need to hide away, to be ashamed of her body, the weaving of the analysis – the restored fabric of the Gobelins, is my comment – and the design chosen from time to time by herself, as she confirms. But when she comes to the picture there is an abrupt halt, and a step back – a "void." I venture a suggestion: the transparency and freedom, which had been achieved through the crystal corridor (long and narrow like the one leading to my consulting room) might show that, in her self-portrait, she had for the time being excluded sexuality from her life. Arms and breasts had been recovered, but legs and genitals were excluded from view, were left unrepresented. *Cupid and Psyche* were there at first, but they disappeared from the scene.

Silence, and then: "I don't agree with any of that, let's change the subject."

I reply, "Of course, change the subject by all means. What do you think of that picture?"

"Nothing, I told you: a picture." After a long silence that I feel as a weight on me, she adds, "The L-shaped corridor makes me think of L for liberty, which I don't have any of."

One of Carine's last dreams.

"I'm sitting with my mother on a strange sofa made of two peninsulas that aren't completely joined but they're so close that I can put an arm around my mother, a calm and affectionate hug. We're watching television, which is actually a screen showing a series of photos from our life. The pictures are moving, not like in a film, but like a 'presentation' with slides of the kind you programme on the computer. I describe them and comment on them to my mother because she was blind, you know.[36] I don't think I've ever told you that. Yes, the peninsulas are two *chaises longues* finally brought together. I had to bring my mother here so she could be cured with me. For me, the analysis has been a second crossing of the ocean."

I comment, "Certainly, and listening to you I understand that there's a completely new version of your life in the dream since, like Columbus, you have discovered a new land across the ocean."

Possession and abandonment had been the starting point for describing the relationship with her mother as it had been lived. Compared to the other flights, this one apparently became paramount to expel a content which had constantly been withheld from the analysis: a suppressed blindness. It has not been a simple matter to bring to analytic thought something that repeatedly seemed to pop into the mind and then immediately became submerged. From this dream onwards, Carine will be able to re-examine not only her role as daughter to that mother, but her role as a mother with that mother as a model, discovering to her pained surprise the extent to which seemingly normal happenings in fact illustrated her own intrusion into her children's lives, and how her own abandonments were consequences of the excesses of intrusion. Overall, at a moment of possible reconciliation with her sadistic, superegoic parts, she has been able to note that, for all her enormous desire to distance herself from her mother, she was "blindly" repeating her ways of functioning. This very attenuation of sadism, first diluted and then mitigated through analysis, has enabled the patient to take on board this feature of her functioning, and not to punish herself for it but to begin important transformations in her most significant relationships, transformations that were working themselves out over three generations.

Before this, another dream had summed up the working-through of the relationship with the mother and with the masculine, a masculinity which the mother had so denied.

Carine finds herself in a very narrow passageway which opens out onto a riverside where she knows, and hears, that a battle is taking place. Beside her there is an undefined crowd. At a certain point a very handsome young man comes up to her, asks her what has happened, and then suggests walking towards the piazza to see better. When they get there, he picks her up and puts her on his shoulders. She can see better from up there and so she describes the battle as it goes on. At first, she is embarrassed about being in this position, as if she was a little girl, and then she feels uncomfortable: she has just eaten and feels some flatulence building up;

immediately after this she feels great excitement at the rubbing of the man's neck and shoulders against her private parts. When he suggests they eat something together she refuses, telling him she's already eaten, and is angry with herself for saying the opposite of what she really wanted. The man leaves and she feels far away and lost. She shuts herself in an empty, miserable house where she hears the sound of gunfire getting fainter, so she goes outside again and crosses the almost empty piazza hoping to find the young man, but when she is about to cross the bridge, which is a bridge *mid*way between two others, she hears more shooting in the distance, and a woman tells her to be careful because on the other side of the bridge, at *mid*day, towards the *Mezzogiorno*, the south, there is still fighting going on. Undecided, she carries on although she doesn't cross the bridge, and on the other side of the river she glimpses the young man who is now involved in the fighting. She holds back, feeling unable to face the battle, but she understands that the only way to get out of it is to cross the bridge and pass through it. At the end of her account she comments that it is "the only way out of this endless stoppage of time, this endless being outside of time."

The narrow street and the geographical position immediately activate associations about her mother and her relationship with her, dreamed as the indigested meal and the consequent flatulence, together with the need to expel it and free herself from it. This dream seems to summarise in detail the sense of excess, the need for expulsion, first undergone by her and then enacted by her, and the obstructive function in relation to sexuality. In particular, the analytic project of going "*beyond*" is finally clear, getting past the long wade through mud that has accompanied her until that moment, trying to lift herself up to see further, to be clear about the inevitability of separation, the need to cross the bridge which marks the boundary with the conflicted and yet empty area that is her family of origin, but also continuity, "*intermediateness*," the *mid*-way that is the means and the passage, and also the way of *thirdness*, and lastly the need for the passage to be crossable.[37]

Crossable bridges in a discontinuity in the transference

The clinical work recounted in this chapter, along with the transformations it set in motion, aims to portray the unfolding of psychotic defences over several generations[38] without the subject passing through a true psychotic experience, as if the primary objects' most markedly psychotic modes of functioning were spread out on a carpet which has the simultaneous effect of slowing time and of being a still fertile terrain where auxiliary functions can come to the rescue and modify the way time passes. Naturally there can be many variables in play: the different times; the primary objects' modes of functioning; the basic Ego-conditions of the subject which is still being formed; fortunate events that can be exploited as secondary auxiliary functions; and events that instead increase and reinforce the traumatic experience. Much time and much human capital must be expended to deflect an attack on the Ego that was already present at its origin.

All the work of analysis becomes necessary for a reconversion – a vital one, we could say – of the use of time until it becomes possible to attain and use that atemporality which characterises the unconscious. Temporal re-actualisation in the compulsion to repeat, which is a trace of the trauma, is the insult that constantly stymies the Ego and eventually compromises many of its capacities. On the other hand, it is also undeniable that every re-actualisation brings with it a trace of the trauma, a small part that functions autonomously and, thanks to splitting and denial, has accompanied the patient's whole existence. What is also completely visible is how this splitting is never complete and how, in fact, a certain more integrated good functioning has accompanied the Ego in a subterranean manner.

In this way, we rediscover in analytic work a melange of more integrated Ego-functions with others that are still separate and split off, and where the object-investment is compromised. In some cases, however, structural lacks appear, voids that open up chasms over primary and archaic functionings, creating instability in the transference and leading to the discontinuity I noted earlier.

In any case, it remains difficult to determine in retrospect the scale of the early damage that was undergone, since it too consists of multiple and heterogeneous factors. The wounded subject may come to feel a profound narcissistic disappointment, but may also come to be partially deconstructed, left with historical and functional voids because the Ego, whose development proceeds as best it can on other fronts, does not find the unified fabric of a historical continuity to identify with and rely on so that it can integrate these functions in a more or less harmonious manner.

The quantitative diversity of traumatic origins leads to quantitative and qualitative situations in clinical work that are quite different from one another and not always amenable to diagnostic frameworks which evaluate the scale of the damage and the temporal importance of the moment in which they occur. The Ego's structural weaknesses and the conditions in which auxiliary functions can operate so that the Ego may rely on them in a moment shot through with trauma – and again in subsequent moments – are important elements in characterising the differences. Indeed, they are elements that participate singly or in concert in the analytic work of reconstruction, reparation, and renewal of the distorting functions and thus also in a work of re-signification.

Addressing discontinuity in the transference inevitably leads me to re-examine clinical work in the light of the "central phobic position" because I would like to echo André Green's thinking about this clinical feature which he has so carefully described (Green 1998, pp. 5–33).

By "central phobic position" Green means a basic psychic disposition that is generally found in the treatment of certain borderline states. And the adjective "central" is employed to underline how fundamental this feature is in the mental functioning of these cases. What would be examined in analysis would not only be the access to consciousness by certain parts of the analysand's unconscious but rather the resonances and threatening correspondences between certain themes that derive from the repressed; all of which arises not only because of the Superego's sanctions but also through defects in the organisation of the Ego. This would bring about a need to prevent the full development of these contents in the conscious. Some themes which punctuate the subject's history would be mutually reinforcing, not simply by addition but by amplifying each other in a reciprocal evocative contact. This would have an impact on psychic functioning, stopping not only the return of what is oldest and deepest, but also the expansion that ties the themes together.

It is quite clear from this that clinical work does not only involve an attempt to stop the trauma returning; rather, the avoidance of trauma attempts to stop the emergence of relationships which would result in a distressing invasion by uncontrollable forces that are traumatic in themselves, making them even more traumatic. The invasion would in fact have a resonance that amplifies an already intolerable violence.

Hence the idea of a centrality understood as located "between two waters" (a *middle* earth?): a level into which the associative current flows and which, in conflict with the current, obstructs its progress both towards the surface and towards the depths. The object is invariably implicated in this "centrality." Even though the object in question is the analyst and the avoidance impacts on the analytic function as a distinct object – more indeed than on the analyst – the patient fears a state of non-separation between subject and object. The transference onto the analyst is feared because – by means of projection – it would bring to light such a great power of penetration into the patient's thoughts that it would not leave other solutions open. So it becomes necessary to scrub away any communication with the potential for comprehensibility (see Carine's rejection of how I interpreted the dream of her portrait, the long silences in sessions, and my frequent feeling that I was in a fog that obliterated boundaries). The avoidance sets a trap with no way out, and this may create a fear that the analyst will fall victim to the imprisoning situation produced by the patient.

I am returning to the concepts of intrusion and abandonment because they offer a bi-chromatism which characterises all the pathological situations I have tried to re-examine.

Abandonments and flights were often evident in their transferential repetitions as re-actualisations of the manifest trauma. By contrast, the intrusion was present at more subterranean levels and initially less ostentatious.

Via reaction formations in response to the invasiveness experienced with the primary objects, many patients were cooperative and rigorous for a long time in their respect for the setting, but over time it emerged that this attentiveness was an imitative reproduction and the processes of symbolic identification could get no purchase on it. There was often a seductive proposition which repeated the maternal seduction in the transference and resulted in a strong idealisation of the analysis (the idealising and sanctioning Superego), later mitigated over years of analytic work through gradual access to reality-testing which scaled down the idealisation to something more reasonable. Nonetheless, on a countertransferential level I could tell that even this kind of scaling down, recorded as the result of an analysis that was going well, preserved a residue of seductive eagerness to please. Intrusion was not only enacted but naturally also desired as repeating the experience of primary passivity, and was most evident in response to the analyst's silences.

I believe it is important to return to this concept of intrusion in its representational aspect as well.

In cases like this, one possible hypothesis is that there is in fact no void but an intrusive representational trace. For this reason, following Green's hypothesis about the framing structure – the representation of the absence of representation – we could speculate that the screen remains only partially empty and so any subsequent distorting attempt at representation on this screen may fail.[39]

This theoretical viewpoint shifts the way we look at the binomial *trauma-loss* and allows a complementary view by introducing another binomial: *absence-intrusion*.

Using this *binocular vision* we can consider traumatic loss not only as a lack, something diminished, but as something that irrupts *as its lack*, coercively imposes itself, and thus prevents the work of mourning and the recovery of the memory as psychic deformation first and transformation afterwards.

Further reworking some theoretical perspectives visited previously in clinical work, I would say that all this led the analyst to settle into that tangential position – parallel to the analytic process in the long phases of stalemate. This settling also made possible a later, more incisive movement, perpendicular to the process – by means of interpretation – when discontinuity is replaced by a transferential continuity between object and word, and when patients reactivate the possibility of a libidinal investment that oscillates between the object and the Ego.[40]

I think that in these cases the analytic function made it possible to discover a *re-found object* which on the one hand limited itself to indicating the repetitions as protracted necessities for survival, but on the other hand continued to sustain investments in the functions of the Ego through dreaming and then by tying together phantasy scenes that were completely impossible in the early days of treatment.

As I write I have been wondering whether to let this part of the analytic transference-countertransference work be backlit by the clinical case study reconstructed around a single character, or give it a separate treatment of its own. I preferred the first solution.

In fact, this dual trace, *light/backlight*, lends support to my way of understanding the countertransference as work done in dialogue with the transference and hence inevitably composite: work on the *stain* (the dirty linen mentioned by Freud) and work on the *imprint*, the trace of thought and its setting-in-motion, prompted by strong sensory residues of listening.

The text has been traced onto this listening and has sought to articulate itself within its own temporal complexity.

In fact, the countertransference has a diphasic temporality: sudden, abrupt moments sometimes synchronous with what is happening in the session, where the analyst has mobilised multidirectional energies; and diachronous moments when it is possible to rework and refresh these movements, keeping at bay and even directing the impulses, but above all interrogating them, since interpretations will be richly impregnated with this work between interlocutors. I will try, though inevitably not completely, to identify the transition, focusing on certain points which nevertheless cannot be considered separate and existing in a precise temporal sequence since they have always fallen into the diphasic temporality of the countertransference and are recursively integrated.

The acceptance of the transferential weight – the expression, for example, of re-actualised relations with a maternal that excluded the masculine – and the acceptance of an idealised transformative possibility could both be the analyst's own stains if they are only lived in one direction and not in terms of conflict and dialogue, a dialogue in which the analyst knows their role as the one inducing the transference.

Working through the countertransference was a clinical rerun of the difficulties previously faced by the patient who, in the dream of the flood, provided the theoretical elaboration of her own analysis. In this way she refreshed a libidinal investment in the object while being able to maintain a distance to shore herself up against every intrusive, expropriating past desire for the other that might set up camp inside her. The sadistic impulses were reined in, saving their energy from being wasted and letting them be enlisted for constructive experiences.

Recognising a discontinuity in the transference may allow the countertransference a long moment of diachronic time to work it through but it offers no immunity against setbacks in understanding this discontinuity and its untranslatability. Emotional and mental closeness to very difficult patients does not in itself guarantee a continuity for working through the countertransference. There is an ever-present limit to translatability, a limit which no dialogue, however good, will ever surpass.

A human being can come about anywhere, in the most irresponsible manner and with no proper reason at all, but not a passport... You could say disorder is when nothing is in the right place. Whereas order is when the right place has nothing in it.

(Berthold Brecht, *Refugee Conversations*, 1940)

Notes

1 Her compelling theory of psychosis marks an invaluable advance in the history of psychoanalysis but, precisely because it was naturally not the only one to address the subject, it may be enriched by a theoretical heritage that remains current. Concepts of partiality, heterogeneity, relationship with the maternal object, phantasy, pleasure and desire, thinking, etc. recur, together with wholly original ideas and concepts such as the pictogram, the primal process, metabolization, word-bearer. The author's rich range of theoretical complementarity enabled her to extend and deepen her metapsychological approach to the psychic structures being examined, as well as paying very close attention to the relationship with the mother, to otherness in general, and to the transgenerational relationship in particular, leaving a theoretical legacy we cannot do without because of the indispensable way it reinforces the therapeutic approach. I will return to some of these concepts in Chapter VII.

2 The emphasis in italics is intended to indicate, in a visual and schematic summary, how such un-homogeneous factors may contribute to the complexity of the original theories about trauma, as they do to later ones, for the avoidance of any temptation to a facile reading of the evidence. This complexity also gives us a reason for the difficulty encountered by Freud in his theoretical treatment of trauma, especially in reconnecting the cardinal points of his metapsychological thinking about instinctuality and phantasying.

3 I am referring to the Weissian concept of *destrudo*, which is taken up in Freud's second drive theory in the concept of the death instinct. On this see also Rita Corsa, *Edoardo Weiss a Trieste con Freud*, 2013.

4 See also Freud S., *The Complete Correspondence of Sigmund Freud and Karl Abraham: 1907–1925*, 2002.

5 On the concept of splitting in Ferenczi see also the paper read by Jorge Luis Martin-Cabré at the seminar held at the Florence Centre of Psychoanalysis, entitled "Trauma, primitive traces, and transference"

(2 October 2021). Also Martin-Cabré J.L., *Autenticità and reciprocità: un dialogo con Ferenczi*, 2016.

6 I would also invite the reader to dwell for a moment on the gruff Freud's tender side by referring to film footage that shows him with a little girl, giving her a flower picked in Marie Bonaparte's garden in Vienna. (The photo of this scene, taken from the film, was shown at the conference *Da Narciso a Lady Gaga* held in Pisa on 25 November 2012.)

7 Carine's "*petrified*" is a projective expression indicating the abolition of her internal perception, an abolition that probably intervened very early in her life. Her description of her mother's conduct as intrusive, demanding, de-subjectivating, and dominant leads me to think of Medusa and her petrifying gaze. The reference in theory is to an excess of perception by the child who, being mirrored in the mother's gaze, cannot enact that exchange which, in good circumstances, becomes a structuring return. A demanding, intrusive gaze bringing an excess with it annuls or amplifies the perceptual elements of the *infans*, petrifying self-perception and hence the potential for self-representation.

8 A for analyst and P for patient.

9 A recurring image in traumatised patients.

10 The *bad enough* mother adapts Winnicott's expression about a *good enough* mother. Reaching adequacy, even in badness, would seem like an achievement in a history where the excesses border on the indescribable. The disorganising excesses in a young life often seem the first thing to be scaled down in clinical work, but in the countertransferential working-through with these patients, the good and the bad are kept at bay as continual risks of increased splitting, precisely because of this tendency to disorganising excess.

11 An expression used by Lacan to describe the birth of the subject. The other's gaze reflected in the mirror is an interesting image of Freud's *primary narcissism*, as Lacan himself acknowledged, which is perhaps also suggested by the game that little Ernst played with himself in the mirror rather than with the cotton-reel.

12 In *Playing and Reality* (1971) Winnicott claims that the mother's face, and I would add her gaze, is the precursor of the mirror. In *Le discours mélancolique* (1993), Marie-Claude Lambotte envisages a fully elaborated traumatic situation in the subject's first contact with exteriority. Referring back to the Lacanian hypothesis of the subject's identification with the image in the mirror where the subject and the Other appear, Lambotte pictures this identification in melancholy as

being based on a pre-mirror situation where exteriority functions as primal cause and as traumatic model. Thus she envisages a pre-mirror order in which the object, not yet identified, is pure exteriority that offers no satisfaction. The subject, identifying with the nothing, loses the illusion of the encounter with the object and falls into a compulsive rejection where the affirmation of the lack stops him attributing any value to the object. And so this condition prevents his own image from being registered within a frame, creating the tragic functioning of the "Ego outside the frame" where the Ego and the other are left killed.

13 Following a different theoretical line of thought, Bion's *rêverie*, we can say that in this case the mother's thinking function was missing as a capacity for *alpha* function that should have offered structural support. Naturally this trauma, which should be understood as occurring earlier than the trauma inflicted on the body, may have partial consequences, as is demonstrated by the fact that many patients, like Carine, can develop remarkable capacities for psychic and intellectual functioning in some spheres but are never able to "link" their emotional experiences to these. See also Bion's "Attacks on linking" (1959) and Green's work on *déliaison*.

14 Porciatti V., Ventura L., "Retinal ganglion cell functional plasticity and optic neuropathy: A comprehensive model," *Journal of Neuro-Ophthalmology*, 2012.

15 This concept will be addressed at greater length in the next section, *Theoretical, clinical, and methodological reflections*, to highlight its applicability to treatment.

16 As in the previous note, this concept will be more extensively addressed in the next section, *Theoretical, clinical, and methodological reflections*. For now, however, I want to point out that the term "curfew," inflated in meaning since the protective restrictions caused by Covid-19, was used for the first time by me in the expression "narcissistic curfew" (*couvre-feu narcissique*) in an article published in the *Revue Belge de Psychanalyse* (2015) entitled *Le trauma et le temps autobiographique*.

17 See also: Denis A. ("Temporality and modes of languages," *International Journal of Psychoanalysis*, pp. 1109–1119, 1995a, and again in "Le present," *Revue Française de Psychanalyse*, pp. 1083–1091, 1995b, which Green cites in *Le temps éclaté* (translated into English as *Time in Psychoanalysis: Some Contradictory Aspects*).

18 On the potential for any containing function to act transformatively on the structuring of the Ego, cf. the concept of *envelope* which René Roussillon reworks from Anzieu's *le Moi peau* (see, among others,

Roussillon R., "L'oggetto coppia," *Psicoterapia e scienze umane*, 48, pp. 289–300, 2014).

19 Segre L., *Sopravvissuta ad Auschwitz* [Survivor of Auschwitz], 2005. Segre L., Palumbo D., *Fino a quando la mia stella brillerà* [Until my star shines], 2018.

20 Prete A., *Compassione. Storia di un sentimento*, 2013.

21 *Exodus* 12, 26–27. The sacrifice of Passover (*Pesach*) is when the Lord passed over (*pâsâchti*) the houses of the Israelites in Egypt, sparing them.

22 To Antonio Prete's concept of "belonging to oneself" I would add "belonging to being," with a cross-reference to Chapter VII, "Crossing Time: Historical temporality in psychotic potentiality."

23 *Stalker* (1979) is based on the book *Roadside Picnic* by Arkady and Boris Strugatsky. "The Zone is life. Passing through it, man is either broken or resists. If he resists, it will depend on his sense of his own dignity and his ability to distinguish the fundamental from the transitory," Tarkovsky said in an interview, and he went on: "What we call passions are not spiritual energy but only friction between the spirit and the outside world." The often wordless film describes a slow journey in the Zone, to which entry is forbidden because it is so dangerous. The three protagonists are a writer, a professor, and the stalker, their illegal and ambiguous guide. He is a former physicist, fallen on hard times and involved with the criminal underworld, but an expert on the prohibited territory. He guides them to the Room, which the writer wants to enter to recover his inspiration while the professor wants to win the Nobel Prize. In this threatening, completely disorienting, and always misty scenario of uncertain boundaries, and sometimes none at all, three different conceptions of life collide with one other: weakness and strength, flexibility and rigidity, hardness-dryness and freshness. The film was made in Russia, still the Soviet Union, which allowed Tarkovsky to return from exile. Some scenes were shot in Estonia and Tajikistan, both then in the USSR. I would like to point out that besides the trauma of exile – though it was voluntary – Tarkovsky's life also contained the trauma of abandonment by his father when he was thirteen years old.
The adventurous journey and the importance of the guide are key elements in Akira Kurosawa's 1975 film *Dersu Uzala*, which will be cited in chapter 7.

24 Bollas C., *The Shadow of the Object: Psychoanalysis of the Unthought Known*, 1987 (see also n32 in Chapter 7).

25 To link my theory with these other perspectives, it could also be said that the theoretical image of *possessing the trauma* would already include

within it a transformation into *alpha* offered by the analyst. However, this is merely an attempt at translation.

26 Kris Ernst, "Ego psychology and interpretation in psychoanalytic therapy," *Psychoanalytic Quarterly*, 1, 15–30, 1951. In *The Psychoanalytic Study of the Child*, vol. 1–25, 1975.

27 In this theoretical context I want to recall Elvio Fachinelli and his revisiting of psychic temporality, and in particular the meaning of *repetition*.

Fachinelli proposes a *propulsive idea of repetition* which is nothing like an eternal return of the same thing, as the compulsion to repeat has often been understood and as it is frequently attributed to Freud. When he talks about the paradox of repetition, Fachinelli contrasts what he calls a *pessimistic view of repetition* recognisable in Kierkegaard, and also he says in Freud, proposing a view that is, if anything, more Heideggerian (cf. *Being and Time*). For Fachinelli, the "*ripresa*" is in fact a *re-presenting of the past* which does not undergo an impoverishing reductionism but *puts life back into action*, opening it up to confirmation or modification. The subject becomes responsible for their repetition, for their refusal to move forwards, or alternatively for their commitment to overcoming the problem. The overcoming of repetition thus acquires an ethical valence. Although his theoretical position is decidedly different from the one I am proposing, both in its theoretical and clinical significance and as a metapsychological derivative on which I have drawn for the notions of *possessing the trauma* and *narcissistic curfew*, it was incumbent on me to recall it for several reasons, and two in particular. First, because he was an unforgettable, though controversial, psychoanalyst and theorist, and secondly because his concept of repetition, for all its difference from mine, sheds light on a progression-in-becoming (cf. Fachinelli E., "Nuovo significato del disegno e recupero magico del passato nell'opera di un'artista psicotica," 1964; Fachinelli E., *Il bambino dalle uova d'oro*, 1974; Benvenuto S., *La "ripresa" estatica di Elvio Fachinelli*, 2011).

28 In relation to this, I note that in *Agonie, clivage et symbolization* (1999), René Roussillon deals at length with trauma, devoting much space to the question of the object's survival in traumatic situations, but he prefers a different diagnostic outlook. He focuses his discussion on what he calls *narcissistic sufferings of identity* associated with non-symbolic primary links, which nevertheless leaves room for considerable fuzziness between different diagnostic approaches.

29 See Pontalis J.-B., *Entre le rêve et la douleur* (1983). Here he maintains that one does not become an analyst without going through psychic

pain, but also that one does not continue to be an analyst – in my preferred translation, one does not *remain* an analyst – without going through physical and psychic pleasure.

30 See Bion W.F., *Learning from Experience* (1962); *Transformations: Change from Learning to Growth* (1965); "A theory of thinking" in *Second Thoughts* (1967).

31 See also his *Standing in the Spaces: Essays on Clinical Process, Trauma, and Dissociation* (1998).

32 Roussillon R., *Agonie, clivage et symbolisation* (1999).

33 The disorganisation was seeking and finding an order that tidied it up by trying to bring it together without "tying it down." Using a Bionian theoretical approach we could perhaps say that the K links to knowledge were being challenged by anti-links (-K). If we follow Green's approach, which is not antithetical to Bion's, there was a lack of *liaison function* to foster the mind's *thirdness function*, a thirdness that is not an alternative to primary and secondary process but, on the contrary, is both the precondition of the transition from one to the other and also integrated with, and constantly present in, the exchange. Green finds many opportunities to emphasise the need for this function and describes the lack of it in psychotic situations where it is not true to say that the secondary process is totally lacking. Rather, what are lacking are the tertiary transitions which would be the intuitive and creative functions linked to emotional situations that are very close to primary functioning but capable of abstraction. This is why, in these situations, he suggests that the analyst lend their own mind's thirdness functions to assist the patient in rehabilitating theirs, always assuming these functions are not coming into being for the first time. As is well known, the concept of thirdness is taken up again by Ogden but with a different, intersubjectivist approach. For Ogden, the third is created and constructed in the analytic field between the thought-functioning of patient and analyst: it is a third subject.

34 Once again, see *revêrie* in Bion; *mirroring–attunement* in Winnicott; and Piera Aulagnier's *violence of speech* which imposes meaning.

35 At-one-ment?

36 The mother had been affected by a serious condition that left her almost blind from an early age, but there had been silence about this fact in the analysis until now, just before its conclusion: a petrifying blindness in the gaze fixed on the daughter.

37 A passage from the sacred Hebrew text, the *Talmud*, recalls that bridges are important but, if they are to be true ways of communication, they

must be low enough to be crossed without fear. *Talmud* means "study," but in fact it collects a series of rabbinical comments and opinions on the ethical, judicial, and ritual rules of the Jewish people and the *aggadah* (examples, parables). The text is open in nature. It dates from the third century BCE and has been translated into English, and only partly into other languages.

38 For an observation on transgenerational psychotic defences, and especially for an assessment of the exclusion of the masculine and the paternal that is often associated with these, see Chapter VII.

39 Green puts forward a similar hypothesis about the *dead mother* complex, speculating that the trace of the maternal imago, which coalesces the two parental figures, persists into adult life.

40 Following Freud's *On Narcissism: an Introduction* (1914), I have tried to develop the features of a good narcissistic withdrawal in Breccia, *Narciso e gli Altri* [Narcissus and the Others] (2014).

III

RITUALS AND REPETITIONS

The theme of this chapter moves temporarily and partially away from clinical practice to enter the history of anthropology and religions in search of the roots of rituals and repetitions.

I am not following this path solely because I want to move beyond the idea of a transgenerational transmission in the form of phantasies of something primitive linked to origins, but also to engage in dialogue with other disciplines which have specific interests in this sphere of knowledge so that our encounter may open new horizons of reflection and new mirrorings for representing the obscure, intense, and sometimes disturbing traces linked to both the origin and the conclusion of life.

From the history of religions to anthropology

It is interesting to reveal the etymological derivations of these two terms – ritual and repetition – considered similar and sometimes used almost as synonyms, and yet absolutely not identical or interchangeable, as is testified by their etymons, both derived from Latin.

Ritual places the weight of the etymon on the prefix *ri-* which indicates "flow," "proceeding towards."

Repeat derives from the Latin *rĕpetĕre* and consists of a prefix *re-*, "once again," but also simply "reinforce, strengthen," and a second part, *petĕre*, "ask, put into words."

DOI: 10.4324/9781003747581-4

I wanted to point out the etymological roots of the two terms to emphasise how, in relation to action and temporality, active and passive features are co-present in them both.

They are clearly two terms in motion, but seemingly in opposite directions: one aiming at advancing towards, flowing further, while the other seems to reinforce a question, a going back to ask again, a return to something already known rather than a movement towards a becoming. In our customary usage, however, the sense of "the passive," "the always equal and identical," seems to attune itself with these terms, altering their meaning, but above all, homogenising them, leaving them undifferentiated so that they become, if not synonyms, then at least terms that fall into the same temporal and functional sphere: that which is always the same, conservative, unvaried.

This teaches us how the common use of language sometimes disfigures the lexical sense of language itself, and this transformation, like others, is neither positive nor negative but merely a source of curiosity.[1]

So in this case as in many others, going back to origins can help us follow its path.

Every ritual can in any case be individual as well as group or collective, and the repetitions of obsessional disturbances indicated by the term "ritualised behaviour" recall this: but ritual, which also expresses a sacred function – that out of which it was born – has an end and a participation almost as extensive as the entire collective.

Among the anthropologists who have addressed these aspects of human behaviour in an attempt to elaborate a general theory of ritual there are many who have concluded that the enterprise was futile and indeed risky because of the varied and multidimensional nature of the historical situations and human behaviours involved in it. Despite this, much has been written about ritual both by anthropologists and by historians of religion, and so a range of different paths have inevitably been followed in defining its forms and contents.

It is to James Frazer, a British anthropologist from the second half of the nineteenth century, that we owe the idea of ritual consisting in an action founded on magical-religious, not scientific, beliefs. In the history of theories about ritual, Frazer has had a wide following for his "intellectualist" theory, as it has been called, and opened up a truly vast field of reading for Freud, a field in which Freud was already interested because of his passion for objects from the ancient world. Frazer's book *The Golden Bough* (1890) undoubtedly had a profound impact on Freud and influenced many of his writings.[2]

Before *Mourning and Melancholia* of 1915a, a completion of the *Papers on Metapsychology* (1915b), the subject of mourning had already been addressed by Freud in *Totem and Taboo* (1913) from an anthropological viewpoint. Freud had indeed been a highly enthusiastic reader of *The Golden Bough*, and Frazer's documentary evidence aroused extraordinary interest at the time, so that the book was translated into many languages and went through forty editions between 1890 and 1915. It was really *a study of mourning*, as is evidenced by the various rituals present in humanity since the most distant times; rituals which, though occurring in different times and places, have maintained certain common features.

Since Frazer, as Vito Lattanzi recalls in his study "Azione rituale, simboli culturali e storia" [Ritual action, cultural symbols, and history],[3] ritual has on the whole been evaluated differently, from a viewpoint thoroughly alien to the opposition between religion and science. According to this approach, termed "functionalist" or "symbolist," ritual would be an instrument endowed with a symbolic efficacy entirely devoted to governing a certain social order, and should therefore be considered a means both of regulating interpersonal relations and of defining the nexuses between nature and society (Simonicca and Dei, *Simbolo e teoria nell'antropologia religiosa* [Symbol and theory in the anthropology of religion], 1998). Situating himself on a different interpretative plane, Vittorio Lanternari (*Festa, carisma, apocalisse* [Festival, charisma, apocalypse], 1983) recognised in ritual the co-presence of sociological and psychological elements side by side, holding that in this way the unconscious dimension of the ritual process can also be understood. Other authors have primarily endorsed the communicative aspects of any ritual celebration, without forgetting the creative features, while still others have reified ritual in order to underline the constant opposition between the rational and the irrational. In the twentieth-century literature, to cite Lattanzi (2000) again, it finally became possible to acknowledge the difficulty of clearly distinguishing between "ritual" and "non-ritual" actions, precisely because of the extraordinary quantity of viewpoints from which this subject can be addressed.

The actions and strategies of ritual thus seem to evade any precise conceptualisation; and this is regardless of the many theories about ritual.

The area of greatest interest for the present study is its relationship with repetition.

Cyclical returns

Cyclical returns in the history of religions are addressed at length by Raimon Panikkar in *Divinità* (2007, with an introduction by Brunetto Salvarani),[4] a volume in which he makes a deep examination of the phenomenology of divinity, starting from Anaximander, for whom everything goes back to the *ápeiron*.

With regard to the origins of the cyclical returns present in the most ancient religions, mostly in reference to the cosmos, there is recurrent reference to the *ápeiron*. And yet it should be remembered that the philologist Semerano (*L'infinito: un equivoco millenario – Le antiche civiltà del Vicino Oriente e le origini del pensiero greco* [The infinite: a thousand-year misunderstanding – the ancient civilisations of the Near East and the origins of Greek thought], 2001) specifies that the word *ápeiron* has distant origins in the Semitic *ápar* (dust, earth), the Akkadian *eperu*, and the Biblical *áfar*, and also recalls that in Greek, *épeiros* (Doric *ápeiros*, Aeolian *áperros*) indicates the earth and mud. According to Semerano all these terms correspond to *ápeiron*, "which was given the neuter article *tò*, sign of confusion" (2001, p. 32). The fragment of Anaximander, which has always been translated as "*first is the infinite*," should therefore be read as "*the first of things is the earth.*" Essentially, all things derive from dust and make their return to it, a concept which recalls the Biblical message of *Genesis* where God says to the man, "Dust thou art and to dust thou shalt return." In terms of the idea of repetition, a repetition aimed at an eternal return, Semerano's valuable philological discoveries have left their mark on the idea of return, and changed its meaning. It was unthinkable that they should be omitted.

Semerano writes:

> From time immemorial, since around twenty-three centuries ago, the cultural world of the West has been challenged by that term, *ápeiron*, which the ancient Milesian thinker laid down as a large, rugged rock to seal his work *On Nature*; and it is more than

> a boundary stone: it is the viaticum from eternity to the void. His successors, who understood it to mean "limitless," "infinite," translated the philosopher's ancient faith in the infinite motherhood of the Earth who waits to receive into her breast what she herself has produced.
>
> (2001, p. 56)

Every civilisation contains the conception of the end and beginning of a temporal period founded on the observation of cosmic rhythms, in a system of periodic purifications and cyclical regeneration of life and time. At the end of each year a past concludes, marking the time that has gone by. The ceremonies of purification are thus bearers of a meaning which absolves the guilts of the individual and the collective through a new birth, in an attempt to restore the pure time of creation: in every new year the cosmogony is repeated. In this view of things, time thus assumes a cyclical movement towards *the eternal return*.

The reason for *the eternal return* is clearly present in *Greco-Roman culture*, in whose philosophical and religious thought, according to Panikkar (2007), an antihistorical stance can be detected, almost a *defence against History* and a sort of counter-offer of *static becoming*, with a consequent annihilation of time's reversibility.

In the Iranian and Judaic religions, however, the duration of the cosmos was limited to a certain number of millennia. History can nevertheless be annihilated and abolished several times before the final *éschaton*. Therefore, Panikkar and Salvarani (2007) hold that doctrines about the cosmic cycles constitute a way that the human being has found to *tolerate History*.

And indeed for psychoanalysts, in particular for those who have always worked with psychosis, it is not at all difficult to understand this resistance, this desire-necessity to flee from History because it is shot through with destructive acts to such an extent that pieces of the story are missing: a desire for flight which sometimes causes injuries that are worse than traumatic, a fact to which the various denialisms of our time provide new testimony.

Panikkar reveals a common feature of these Hellenistic-Oriental doctrines, one characterised both by the way it punctuates the given historical moment, causing the present to seem decadent compared to previous periods of history, and the way it brings to light signs of an incipient regeneration. In the end, *History is borne because it is necessary for future regeneration*. Rome had two fundamental myths: *the life of the City*, limited to a certain number of years, and the *Great Year*, which marked the end of Rome's history in the final *ekpyrosis*. The reign of Augustus repeats the *Golden Age*, a mythical time of prosperity and abundance described first by Hesiod (*Works and Days*, eighth century BCE) and sung again by Virgil in the *Georgics* (42 BCE–39 BCE) to indicate the return to a *new Golden Age* which confirms the cyclical view of History but one that cannot do without the descriptions of wars and epidemics which become signs of transition, and thus are no longer warning signs indicating a transition to come but the real passing from one age to the next: a sort of renewed attempt at valorising History.

Christian thought completely transcends these schemata of eternal repetition by instead emphasising the importance of personal renewal. This is testified by the thinking of St Augustine (354–430 CE), for whom the idea of God enabled the recognition of unified design and divine will in human events. So History becomes the product of human wills guided by a supreme Authority and thus the followers of cyclicality and dualism are shown their error: that of starting from a false conception of reality because they do not properly know the essence and possibility of mankind. "Historiography, *historia*, then becomes, for St Augustine, a narrative literary genre of things that really happened while historical facts, the *res gestae*, are named with special attention to temporal expressions such as *spatia temporum*, *volumina saeculorum*, *contextus ordo saeculorum*, to indicate the movement, development, and connection between historical events and a temporal succession that indicates mutability.... Therefore he did not admit any historical scepticism."[5] "Things that are past do not themselves exist, but only certain signs of them as past, the sight or hearing of which makes it known that they have been and have passed away" (*De Trinitate*, XIV, 8). Augustine thus animates history through the *ambivalence of time*.[6,7]

The archaic conception of time becomes archetypical and antihistorical, and is gradually distinguished from the modern, post-Hegelian conception. The historicist perspective can thus enable humanity to bear the pressures of History.

The name of Hegel reminds us that he valorises the historical event in itself through the concept of *historical necessity*, which justifies sufferings by the necessity of the "historical moment" and, according to Panikkar, we can find in this a connection to the

Judaeo-Christian conception. In fact, Hegel sees History as the coming and manifestation of the universal spirit, like God, and repetition of thesis–antithesis–synthesis, unlike Marx, who completely strips History of transcendent meanings as the epiphany of the class struggle.

The antihistorical horizon cannot, however, be superseded within the historicist perspective itself, as Salvarani writes in the introduction to his 2007 text, but is superseded, for the first time in history, by the Judaeo-Christian religion which introduced a new category: faith, or creative freedom for the man who leans on God. Faith can attribute trans-historical meaning to historical tragedies. While archaic man was opposed to History because he found himself to be powerless in the face of his own suffering and natural catastrophes, and thus attributed it all to magical and demoniacal influences, the Prophets instead interpreted calamities as negative or positive theophanies. For the first time, according to Salvarani, the Prophets valorise History, discovering one-way, non-cyclical time, and interpreting it as the will of God who intervenes in History, which thus becomes a divine epiphany.[8] The monotheist revelation in fact happens in a time with a historical duration (the *Laws of Moses*) and entails the acceptance of History as a continual dialogue with God, as an expression of the need for a strong spiritual striving in mankind.

In Hebrew culture History is conceived in a more limited manner, as a necessity, in the hope that it ceases with the Last Judgement; in the Messianic conception, by contrast, History has an eschatological function in which periodic renewal is replaced by regeneration once only, in the future.

Regardless of any interpretation that sees the anti-historicist period as being concluded, the cyclical theory of time was nonetheless highly durable, lasting until the seventeenth century (as witnessed in the works of Dante, Bacon, Campanella, and Bruno), when a more linear theory of History intervenes, with a faith no longer placed in an *infinite plan* but in *infinite progress*, a faith that runs from Pascal to the Enlightenment.

Even so, the question of cyclical return has still not been definitively abandoned. In 1900, with Nietzsche, the cyclical conception of History and time returns once again. "This life as you now live it and have lived it, you will have to live once again and innumerable times again; and there will be nothing new in it, but every pain and every joy and every thought and sigh and everything unspeakably small or great in your life must return to you, all in the same succession and sequence" (*The Gay Science*, 1882, p. 341). However, Nietzsche's vision of the eternal return differed from that of philosophers from the ancient world in the interpretative use that he makes of the myth. According to a reading of the text proposed by Deleuze (*Nietzsche and Philosophy*, 1962), the return does not belong to being but, on the contrary, constitutes it as an affirmation of becoming and of that which passes and so it is an affirmation of the different or the multiple. Nevertheless, later in *Thus Spoke Zarathustra* (1961 [1883]), Nietzsche reiterates that "all things recur eternally, and we ourselves with them, and that we have already existed an infinite number of times before, and all things with us" (p. 237). And proleptically, without specifically developing concepts about the eternal return, he created the premise for it in *The Birth of Tragedy: or Hellenism and Pessimism* (1872), writing on the recurring return of myth, the Antichrist, a primal force, and a regenerative beauty: an "intrinsically healthy, ancient, and original force lies hidden, which admittedly only stirs itself powerfully at occasional moments of tremendous importance before returning to its dream of a future awakening" (§ 23).

One question comes to the fore in this journey through historical, philosophical, and religious thought: did archaic mankind, but also the archaic part of every human being, repeat in order to save themselves from evil and in doing so exorcise it and become alienated by ahistoricising themselves in a magical perspective? Did the Messianic faith of the Judaeo-Christian religion save humankind by historicising them?

There can be no unanimous responses, human reality being multiple and heterogeneous, bringing with it archaic elements which evil, catastrophe, or injury reactivate through processes of regression, as rediscovered by Freud, so that the trauma re-actualises the previous trauma, going all the way back to the most archaic moments in the life of humankind, laid down transgenerationally and unremembered in every one of us. Thus the responses may be multiple, but many of them try to counter the repeating of the harm.[9]

What have religions taken from all this?

Giovanni Filoramo, Professor of the History of Religions and later of the History of Christianity at Turin University, yet avowedly secular, writes in the introduction to his wonderful book *Il grande racconto delle Religioni* (2018):

> Religions are world-views. This statement refers to how different representations, investments, or hypotheses in a specific field of knowledge draw order and coherence from a central, focal point which provides the master key to a set of knowledges that would otherwise appear jumbled and confused. World-views may be individual or collective. Today, for example, in the triumphant era of religious individualism, it is the prerogative of the individual to construct their own coherent world-view, a sort of compass to help them navigate the sea of life (and above all, the internet...). But for centuries religious world-views were a cultural reality received within the tradition one was born into, which at the very most could be rejected, but certainly not constructed at will. These religious views... collected and crystallised a specific religion's sense of the sacred in mythical stories, cults, ceremonies, ritual practices, artistic and architectural forms. At bottom, they were *the systems of cultural orientation* which made it possible to position oneself in the world, providing guidelines for deciphering the essential questions that assail mankind, guidelines based on fundamental dichotomies like transcendent-immanent, above-below, invisible-visible, uncontrollable-controllable.... In its naked, raw truth, we live today in the condition of mankind prophetically described by Max Weber a century ago: "A feeling of unprecedented inner loneliness of every individual." The gods have abandoned humanity.... And yet religion continues to walk among us. A *revenant*? An empty simulacrum? I don't think so.
>
> (2018, pp. 12–13, italics in original)

The gaze Filoramo casts on the present, the current, actual moment, is provocative and unsettling. In using these terms – present and current – I am not simply indicating an interval of time but also a psychic functioning which, acting further on the action, takes away space for thought, sucks it up, and, in making it present again, sucks up the idea that is linked to the "thing" to represent it.

For Filoramo too, religion has always been a link, a foundation of legitimacy with the cosmos. Time was marked by liturgical rhythms; religion integrated the lives of all, believers and non-believers.

The anthropocentric turn engineered by the Enlightenment, in some ways the child of that same Christianity which brought God so close to man by incarnating Him, threw transcendence into a crisis by placing man and the world on the same level. Now it is science that interprets the world. With the loss of religion as a glue, the world has been secularised according to Filoramo, and yet modernity, which has been an epochal challenge for religions, has also made a contribution to their paradoxical revitalisation. The world of religion returns because it never died: it underwent various metamorphoses and now reappears to fill the voids left by an accelerated, always interconnected, *liquid society* (Zygmunt Bauman, *Liquid Modernity*, 2000) which commercialises religions and dislocates them by making them lose contact with their habitual places. According to Filoramo, we are witnessing a "God who speaks out of context" (Zygmunt Bauman, *Liquid Modernity*, p. 528) and a response to this which is simultaneously an adaptation and resistance to the structural changes, with added fundamentalist and literalist impulses fostered by *nationalistic tendencies which have replaced religions' capacity for an ethical and identitary foundation* (and are perhaps replacing *any* capacity for an ethical and identitary foundation). All of which also leads to exacerbations of individualism such as the "personal God" or "spirituality without God" (p. 529). Nevertheless, like Filoramo, and setting aside the scepticism that inevitably derives from glimpsing the narcissistic freight in all this, I have no doubt that in this jumble of disorganised, and often disorganising, elements, there is a pluralism in religious modernity which, compared to their religions of origin, is returning to a cosmocentrism located in the ecosystem.

In the full awareness that one risks a perverse circularity, a risk present in any circularity that does not introduce changes – as is suggested by Merleau-Ponty's concept of recursion[10] – it is nevertheless important to be able to think that both pluralism and the dualism to which Filoramo refers (between a God who speaks out of context and a personal God) might be *life-rafts* for belief, a belief which, as Paul Laurent Assoun reminds us (*L'Entendement Freudien: Logos et Ananké*, 1984), is the vital part of the *logos* and at the same time a constant threat to it.

Revisiting Filoramo's thought, we may think that religions have maintained in History that impulse to collective aggregation in which the individual is not obliterated, does not wither away, and perhaps has more ways to confront the "personal God" who risks becoming the individual himself. In other words, they seem to have maintained over the millennia that redemptive potential for sharing, participation, and the necessary comparison with the other.

The otherness offered by religions is perhaps supportive, an attempt to combat the paranoid hatred of the other, reducing the deceit of the Ego's narcissism and alienating its omnipotence, so that celebration is no longer that of a crowd celebrating the return of a hero who represents them – in fact a complacent self-celebration in which the hero tries to divert the applause of the multitude onto himself – but a recollection, a memento, and a warning, to which reference can be made and towards which we can return. Not a rituality emptied of meaning but a meaning in a state of becoming, which celebrates continuity with a transgenerational past on which to base new existences.

While Filoramo reminds us how far the modern world has constructed personal divinities without meaning, Chianese in his book *Il Vivente e il Sacro* [The living and the sacred] (2020) emphasizes that the sacred is indispensable to human life, and the term *life* is in tune with his title. He starts out with observations from several palaeontologists for whom the relics of *Homo naledi* represent a family tomb, then adds the prehistorical studies of Jean Clottes (2008) who precedes *Homo sapiens* with *Homo spiritualis* (Chianese, p. 44), coming finally to the conclusion that "this immense transfer from the merely physical to the imaginary… is central to mankind" (p. 46).

Following Bataille (1955), Chianese also stresses that while palaeolithic artists painted animals to abandon their past, "the journeys and descents into chthonic, infernal worlds will continue to be undertaken for millennia, until they arrive at us" (Chianese, p. 47). The "need to believe" (Chianese, p. 192) is therefore primal, original: we can call it a confirmation of what Freud too maintains in *The Future of an Illusion* (1927, pp. 17–18): "man's helplessness (*Hilflosigkeit*) remains and along with it his longing for his father, and the gods."

The land of remorse

In *La terra del rimorso*,[11] Ernesto De Martino addresses the same problem in a very much more restricted environment which foregrounds a collective impulse to aggregation, integrating several disciplines, as do some historians of religion. De Martino looks at these phenomena from a firmly anthropological perspective.

In particular, De Martino found himself studying the relations between migration, deviance, and mental suffering, setting ethnology alongside psychiatry and looking, for example, at the "spellbound" delusions suffered by numerous Italian migrants to Switzerland.

In his head-to-head with Giovanni Jervis, a psychiatrist who was a member of his team, a difference of opinion emerged in every case. For Jervis, the ritual does not save; one must be free in order to be healed, and iteration does not open spaces for any freedom or remission. By contrast, De Martino, who felt a deep pity for the defeated, as is recalled by Clara Gallini in her introduction to his book, finds that the ritual has a role in rescuing sufferers from misery, acting as a *raft*. Here, feeling deeply in tune with De Martino's thought, I want to make a link to the visual symbolism of this by citing Géricault's *The Raft of the Medusa*,[12] a raft which acquires a "symbolic autonomy" (De Martino, p. 23) and, through the "de-historicising of the negative" (p. 22), returns us to the historicism that is necessary in modern research. This is how I will try to engage with these two propositions of De Martino.

His concept of "symbolic autonomy" is a paradox verging on oxymoron. No symbol can be autonomous, by definition, but must express its function by linking itself through synthesis and analogy to the greatest possible number of terms and concepts that can be associated with it and, from a psychoanalytic viewpoint, with a *symbolised unconscious*.

The symbolic autonomy of the *Taranta*,[13] as of the *Tarantato*, the one bitten by the *Tarantula*, who is the central subject of De Martino's studies in Salento,[14] certainly implies the symbolic since it departs from concreteness and works by linking itself to analogy but at the same time is detached from any coherent point of reference.

The drawing of the *Taranta* (spider) which appears in the text as documentary evidence very probably shows *Lycosa tarantula*, "a large, hairy spider, dark in colour, with grey-brown markings on its back and a dark band on a grey-orange background on its belly. Armed with remarkably large chelicerae, its whole appearance suggests the *potency of the bite*, whereas the much more dangerous, but smaller and less conspicuous *Latrodectus tredecimguttatus* does not provoke equally intense emotional reactions" (De Martino , p. 79). From the toxicological point of view, the bite of the former causes a prominent but generally mild local reaction: the exact opposite, we may say, of the second, the *Taranta*. Thus, bite and venom have a meaning that is *symbolic, but autonomous*, detached from the consistency of science. Women are still sometimes given the name *Taranta*, and even *Pizzica* (stinger), passing the dismal legacy on to sisters and daughters.

"The *tarantato*, the person bitten by the *taranta*, dances like a victim possessed by the animal and like a hero who defeats the animal by dancing it": the dance is performed in a striving for "identification" and "agonistic detachment," trying to "let oneself go," "making oneself a spider" and "dancing the spider" (De Martino , p. 83). The *tarantato* submits to its orders, or else takes command, and may come to terms with, or set the date of, the next crisis. But the *Taranta*, its bite and its venom have a symbolic repertoire.

After studying a great many cases, De Martino's team recognised that *il primo morso* (the first bite), a first crisis, corresponds to a psychic trauma, which is followed by a first musical–choreutic–chromatic exorcism. Then comes a series of instances of *ri-morsi* (further bites)[15] fixed in time at intervals established by the tradition of the *Taranta*. De Martino's interpretative hypothesis is that tarantism constitutes a symbolic device by which a conflictual psychic content (for example, a romantic betrayal) which has not found a solution on the conscious level, instead of imposing itself as a psychic symptom, is "evoked and *configured*[16] on the mythical-ritual level, and on this level made to flow away at set intervals, relieving [the subject] of the weight of solicitations in the periods between ceremonies, and facilitating a relative psychic equilibrium during those periods" (De Martino, p. 97).

It seems clear by now that there is an intimate connection between individual psychic drama and collective dramatization in which, as Kaës (*Le Malêtre*, 2012) reminds us, the group helps the individual to bear the traumatically unbearable, but the group is also the concrete and symbolic representation of the transgenerational group identity which preceded both the individual and the group.

As I see it, all of this teaches us not only that ritual has a symbolic autonomy, understood in De Martino's sense, but also that this autonomy may be exponentially multiplied when viewed on the transgenerational plane.

This also allows us to preserve aligned elements outside of time and outside of any rationalist schema, but with salvation as their aim and outcome.

The *ri-morsi* have in fact ended up being established by the *tarantato* in the choreutic-musical group environment, which often coincides with the harvesting of summer fruits, thus leaving time free for life and work: *time redeemed*.

In my opinion, the symbolic autonomy of these ritual events, understood in the transgenerational complexity I have just proposed, appears still more evident in the case of the fifty-year-old countryman described in *La terra del rimorso* (*Le Malêtre*, 2012, p. 99). Pietro was admitted to hospital with a diagnosis of latrodectism which was confirmed during his stay by the medical staff as an advanced state of poisoning. However, as soon as he felt the bite he associated it with the *Taranta* and danced for four days while his audience threw variously coloured ribbons. "The traditional mythical re-enactment in which friends and relations took part, remoulded what had originally been the threads of real historical events into a new form" (*Le Malêtre*, 2012, p. 100).

If we carefully revisit this phenomenon, it seems that there has been no real de-historicising of the events, but that the history of the individual, which sustains itself by being aligned with the history of the group he belongs to, which sustains it in turn, is suspended through arcs of time programmed to give space in which tradition can operate, extending and sustaining the individual and the group with a still wider collective, that of the forebears, the predecessors, the previous generations: ancient, familiar, and alien at the same time. All of this has a thoroughly precise goal: to introduce a redemptive existential individual and group experience and a redemptive temporality.

In the crisis, time stops before beginning again, to give space and time free from crises and evil in which one can work and live. In fact, the dates on which the *morsi* and *ri-morsi* (the first and subsequent bites) fell came during the periods following the summer fruit harvest. Pietro does not obey the stimulus of the venom's toxicity but responds to the embrace of those who came before him and are only symbolically represented by the dancers and musicians.

In fact, what De Martino calls "de-historicising the negative" is *the construction of a time outside historical time, to create a time which in the rite repeats a redemptive temporal potential, so as to reach a time that is indeed redeemed*, and to bring freedom from a traumatic bite of present historical reality to which the single person, and maybe the entire collective they belong to, would be unable to respond with their sole individual resources.

The ritual evokes the presence of forebears, but also performs extraordinary acts of temporal construction and deconstruction, moves out of history, cleanses it of its own negative in order to restore the individual and the group to their own personal and collective history.

The path of the temporal–atemporal–countertemporal entanglement cannot have linear coherence – witness the autonomy of the symbolic invoked by De Martino – but, in my view, it possesses a recursive coherence.

At the end of this process of passing through many expressive modes of temporality, History returns; everything is restored to it, but it has also been transformed.

How much does this experience of anthropological studies refer to the individual psychoanalytic experience which I have called *possessing the trauma*?[17]

Very much indeed, in my opinion. The theories derived from different epistemologies cannot be confused or integrated with each other, still less prove each other, given their high degree of inhomogeneity. Nevertheless, they can meet once more on common ground and draw strength and support from each other.

Perhaps the repetitions we encounter in every clinical case history – for André Green, every symptom is a repetition – are an active, not passive, waiting in search of a *redeemed time.* Perhaps the protagonist is not the death instinct but the daily, compromised, mournful, individual and collective battle with life. A battle with and for life based on the transgenerational burden which aggravates and sustains life by strengthening the identity.

But if it really is the case that every subject, if they are to be alive, must be alive in History, in *Their* history, how could we imagine being treated and cared for outside it?

Since every symptom is a desperate attempt at cure, even though it is often ineffective, repetition is not a flight from History, not a time outside time to stop History, but a time of waiting, a temporal enclave of recovery and crisis, a pause by an Ego hypothecated to a future in which the complex temporal articulation can begin again in continuity with the traumatic experience and with History.

History determines a prospective creation of reality which is nevertheless as indispensable for the individual as it is for the social group and the collective.

As recounted in chapter 2, when Freud's grandson, little Ernst, stops throwing his toys onto the floor to destroy them and wants to preserve the internalised object (his father who betrayed him by going to the war, as well as his mother, who betrays him when she goes away) he develops a game with the cotton-reel so that he can make it reappear whenever he wants. Ernst holds the object *in his power*, and thus preserves and *possesses* it, that object he has constructed by separating the Ego from it during primary narcissism, but it is nevertheless an object that is constructed because it has been fostered by a primal object which historically precedes it. The reel is also endowed with autonomous symbolism and, by making it return, Ernst makes previous history return, de-historicising it before re-inserting himself into it. Thus he gives a bodily, physical, and psychic continuity to the future when, in maturity, having hopefully achieved Ego-equilibrium, belonging will take the place of this possession of the trauma.

In my theoretical representation, by making the cotton-reel return Ernst does not only invoke the return of this father and mother, the predecessors closest to him, but all those who have preceded him over many generations and who, invoked in this way, may bear witness to the trauma of mourning and separation, and give support in it. The anguish about death caused by a frustrating, unwanted separation for which one feels ill-equipped, still incapable, is overcome in the repetitive ritual of the cotton-reel. The object is no longer destroyed, it must be preserved, and can be preserved even if this means using a sleight-of-hand which says less about the child's omnipotence than about the power of the symbol and the community, the group-identity outside the individual which every object represents symbolically along a horizontal line of time.

To my way of thinking, the analyst's work within the analytic process is not about pondering the undecidable question of the historical versus the psychic but about not forgetting their necessary interrelation, as André Green reminds us.

A subject's historical reality, which is suggested as objectified psychic reality and offered to the other, is transformed by the analytic process into new psychic reality where that history is still possible, by valorising the subject who is telling the story, thereby fostering an alternation between the historical and the psychic, sometimes over stretches of time when there is a need for a thoroughgoing reconstruction of missing parts.

In this respect, analytic movement could be considered as the *process of psychicising the historical and historicising the psychic*, in a pendular movement which should permit a continual oscillation between the here and now and the there and then, with a proper balance between them.

The work of mourning

Closely related to what has been said so far is the ancient ritual experience of mourning that I would call work of mourning, as Freud did in *Mourning and Melancholia*, written in 1915a as a complement to, and I would say a completion of, his treatise on *Metapsychology* from the same year, though it would only be published two years later. In this brief, dense draft he expounds the essence of melancholy and compares it with the affective situation of mourning, which is a feeling and not a symptom, until it finds a solution. In this way he separates himself from a more psychiatric perspective, which he had himself embraced in Draft G of 1895, but he stresses that the notion of melancholy has many more features which remain partly obscure.

Once again we encounter Freud's regular methodological plan, which is to clarify a psychopathological phenomenon and set it alongside a so-called normal one. Moreover, this text echoes *On Narcissism: an Introduction* (1914) where he had earlier described melancholic regression and cited Otto Rank's[18] suggestion about the narcissistic basis of object-choice.[19]

In *Mourning and Melancholia* Freud also reprises the theses of Karl Abraham[20] on *cannibal orality* and the *ambivalence of the link* which Abraham speculated were the origin of melancholy. He similarly develops the concept of *identification* (based on Abraham's idea of *incorporation*). Indeed, for Abraham object-love begins between the primitive phase and the late anal-sadistic phase, when there is a reduction in the ambivalence about cannibalistic incorporation conveyed from the second oral phase, that of narcissism, and the dominance of the object begins, understood as aimed at preserving the object itself.

At this point, the sense of guilt, which arises from ambivalence, and the destructive desire to incorporate the object, act with an inevitably traumatic effect which can only be overcome if the value of preserving the object prevails. Otherwise, Abraham observes, a degree of destructiveness may gain the upper hand and lead to depressive disturbance.

However, the central feature of *Mourning and Melancholia* lies in advancing the idea that *work* is done in mourning, according to an economic model similar to that adopted in relation to dreaming.

The definition of *mourning* proposed by Freud is truly vast since, as well as the loss of the beloved person, it includes the loss of all the abstractions that might be equivalent to that person: homeland, freedom, and ideals.

The continuity between pathology and normality which Freud proposes in this text is a fundamental point which recurs in his psychoanalytic theory.[21] It presumes a continuum between pathologies and between pathology and normality, and indicates his openness to new ideas, including those in the sphere of phenomenology which were of great importance at that time. In this book there will be repeated reference to the concept of *continuum*.

Freud anchors himself to a definition of the *psychic economy of mourning*, the loss of interest in the outside world, and the *work of mourning*, operating on the link with the painful memories, to indicate an activity of the Ego that is nothing like a deletion of the memories with the passing of time, even though time is needed for it, as it is in any form of work.

In a word: the work of mourning is not the popular "time heals all wounds."

Instead, in mourning, unlike in melancholy, it is essentially the work of the single subject that enables the object to be "re-found" (or diminished or devalued or declared dead), a work that "deals a death-blow" to death, setting the subject free.

The question of *mourning* had already been addressed by Freud in *Totem and Taboo* in 1913 from a more anthropological viewpoint.

And it is from here that I would like to begin, in order to highlight how the concept of "work" in relation to mourning was implicitly present in humanity from the earliest times in a variety of rituals which, though found in different times and places, have characteristics in common.

The study of anthropology has given prominence to much research on death and funeral rites that is of great interest in differentiating the various geographical regions of Italy.

Among the most famous students of events belonging to nineteenth-century Italian folklore we may recall Giuseppe Pitré (*Biblioteca delle tradizioni popolari siciliane* [Library of popular Sicilian traditions], 1871–1913) and Paolo Toschi (*La poesia religiosa del popolo italiano* [The religious poetry of the Italian people], 1921), who were mostly interested in studying the customs of working people, especially in Southern Italy. In the twentieth century the central figure becomes Ernesto De Martino, cited in the previous section on the *tarantati*, since he made a deep study of the ethnological aspects of popular religion, using investigation in the field and studying the various forms of ritual in a complex and detailed way. The results of his research, and that of his group, are contained in one of his best-known texts, *Morte e pianto rituale nel mondo antico* [Death and ritual lamentation in the ancient world] from 1958.

If culture is an ensemble of intellectual cognitions acquired first by study, experience, and various environmental influences, later re-elaborated in a subjective and autonomous manner, which become a constitutive element of the individual person, it is also true, in a more anthropological sense, that culture is founded on an ensemble of values, symbols, conceptions, beliefs, behavioural models, and various kinds of activity which characterise every social group's way of life. I add this proviso not to emphasise the contents, which are after all rather obvious, but to stress once again the theme of the transformative work behind every attainment.

De Martino's research on the rituality of mourning starts from the idea that human beings, knowing they must die, and in order to overcome this harsh and inexorable element of reality which brings concern and anxiety, try to equip themselves with some anchors for salvation. One of these is represented by the cultural-religious aspect of life, or rather the symbolic creation, by means of life itself, of a wider horizon which may help humankind comprehend and overcome death, so as not to fall prey to madness: that is, the unsymbolisable concreteness which leads to psychic death. It is a work of transformation since the existential aspect of death and life, and their cultural and religious processes, become the continually transformative indicators and revealers of this necessity. At the peak of any suffering, the human being is obliged to pass through the crisis that derives from it, so as not to remain imprisoned in it.

One of the most significant grieving rituals is the *funeral lamentation* whose traces are lost in the mists of time. The *Lucanian traditions*[22] are perhaps the ones that have best preserved the memory of this ancient ritual.

The Lucanian practice of funeral lamentation, and in particular *professional lamentation*, is dying out and all that remains of it are a few vague memories recounted by old women. It is a re-actualisation of very ancient memories, probably pagan in origin, then partly transformed by Christian-Catholic influence in syncretic form as the popular Catholicism that is interwoven with the influence of pagan elements.

The very form of words that are used to portray a death are more pagan than Christian in character. Thus, in the afterlife, the deceased will continue to lead a life not very different from their life on earth: two shirts, one new and one patched, two pairs of underwear, a pipe if he was a keen smoker, and so on.

The whole ritual follows precise *rules* which by tradition construct a *technique of weeping*. The *lamentation* is presented as a text according to models and stereotypes. There are usually no invocations of sacred figures from Christianity: on the contrary, there is almost a kind of protest against them because those remaining alive feel betrayed by death.

The first phase involves the recollection of the deceased, then of his work: for example, the mourner always makes a reference to what the hands of the dead person used to do. Then the memory moves on to the good times. This is followed by a description of the state the family will be left in because of the bereavement: for the bride-to-be a lament for the unconsummated marriage, for the widow the hard task ahead of her, and for the children the absence of their father.

Special importance is attached to what we might call the *mimicking of grief*, as De Martino recalls: the body swaying perfectly in step with the sound, as in a great many African and Amerindian shamanistic traditions, with an almost hypnogenic function very like that of Arabic professional mourners. The mourner's mimicry is embodied in the handkerchief waved over the body of the deceased and then lifted to the nose in a constant repetition of the gesture. This gesture has an atavistic root since it is also found among ancient Egyptian mourners.[23] As De Martino tells us, ritual traditions of this type are still present in other parts of Italy: Sardinia, for example, or Brianza and Valtellina.

In the region around Naples a "*riepito battuto*" used to be performed: a lament accompanied by a ritual of hitting oneself which concluded with some women coming up to the widow, crying "Oh you poor thing!", tearing out a lock of her hair and throwing it onto the body of the deceased.

It was then the custom for the women to go up to the corpse with their hair loose, striking themselves violently on the chest and groaning with grief. The French term for mourning, *deuil*, would seem to illustrate this aspect vividly, deriving from the Latin *dolium* and the associated verb *dolĕre* referring to the beating of the chest.

It was the custom to cut one's flesh, scratch the cheeks and forearms until they bled, to strike oneself, and tear one's clothes and hair (cf. the Rite of Beating).[24]

So these rituals are the atavistic memory of ancient customs. In ancient Greece, for example, we understand from documents and paintings that women with their hair loose came up to the dead person striking their chests. The same tradition is found among the Myrmidons, while in the *Alcestis* of Euripides the god of death is described as brandishing a sword to cut off a lock of the dead person's hair (*Alcestis*, lines 75–78).

Besides displaying genuine grief for the deceased, the whole repertoire of mourning and its gestures seems to conceal an *apotropaic operation* of putting death at a distance, a technique aimed at combatting the *returned of the deceased*, as is testified by other customs, such as burning the dead person's clothes or opening the windows after the death. The interesting phrases that close the funeral lament seem to have the same purpose: in fact, the next of kin reminds the deceased that they have done all they should, that there is no more to be done for them, and invites the deceased to return in a dream and say whether or not they are content with what they have received in funereal honours (as De Martino, 1958, records).

The gestures of mourning are also very much present in the ancient world, as is testified not only in lines of poetry – especially by Homer – but also in figurative art. The reference is to the *Schemata*.[25]

In the figurative art of the ancient world the schemata of mourning are as important as those of adoration (*Ilioupèrsis*). Indeed, the lament for the dead seems to have had remarkable importance in ancient Egypt, where we find all the gestures later used by the Greeks, as recorded in the note about the mourner of Hori (cf. Hans Bonnet, *Reallexikon der ägyptischen Religionsgeschichte*, 1952). The Greeks themselves recognised that their rituals derived from those of Asia, or from the Barbarians, of which there is evidence on some terracotta urns (*làrnakes*) from the Minoan civilisation in Crete (Bronze Age, 2700–1500 BCE). *Làrnax* was the name given to tombs, sarcophagi, and cinerary urns on which we often find women portrayed with their arms raised and scenes of duels leading to the death of the participants.

The female figures have their hands and arms raised above their heads, showing how they beat themselves and tear their hair, a gesture often found later in a highly stylised form as geometric images on the *pròthêsis* – terracotta vessels with representations of funerals and sometimes of *ekphorà*, the transporting of the deceased stretched out on the funeral wagon.[26]

In archaic tombs it is not unusual to find, in addition to urns, statuettes of terracotta adopting this stance, one hand raised above the head and the other on the chest. I recall that Homer also speaks of heroes beating their heads, hips, and thighs as a token of mourning. The gesture of tearing the hair is also well-known from Homer to the Roman era, and is frequently represented on black-figure vases, which also illustrate the scratching of cheeks.

So it is especially interesting to note that what De Martino found by collecting the stories of old women in Southern Italy corresponds very closely to the pictorial evidence of painted urns used in funeral rites from many centuries earlier and a wide range of places in the Mediterranean.

In my view, this multiplicity of times and places goes to support the hypothesis of a powerful need to hand down funeral rites over many generations.

Though the funeral rite, and in particular the gestures of distress, was a prerogative of women, we may note that in the ancient world men also appear in it, as is recorded by the sarcophagus of Tanagra,[27] although their gestures are different.

From the time when black-figure vases were developed, we usually see men raising one or both arms in front of them, a gesture very like that of adoration, and this is probably to be understood as *veneration of the deceased* who is thus *heroized* (Bonnet, 1952). On a black-figure *loutrophòros*[28] in the Berlin Museum all the men are raising their right hand while all the women are striking themselves and tearing their hair. Then, as a sign of the most profound grief, comes the kneeling on the ground, again mostly by the women and accompanied by the other ritual gestures. In our own time the act of kneeling remains associated with the expression of religious testimony.

Among further gestures of mourning, resting the head on a hand is one that embraces a range of feelings and may also signify emotions other than grief. An example of this gesture is portrayed by Exekias (a Greek ceramicist and ceramic painter from 500 BCE) on a *pinax* in the Berlin Museum. (The *pinax* was a small wooden tablet covered in wax which the Greeks used for note-taking and drawing.) The painters of *lêkythoi*, long-necked funerary urns, used this gesture to signify grief, of both the deceased and the bereaved. The reliefs on sarcophagi or on funeral *lêkythoi* with light backgrounds often avoid showing the corpse on the bier; on vessels for ointment the deceased is instead sometimes portrayed on his own tomb in a touching posture of mourning for himself, which I find particularly interesting since it seems to indicate a recovery, in narcissistic terms, of the image of the deceased.

To represent a relatively contained grief on Attic reliefs it is mostly sufficient to show the hands clasped, the head bowed or resting on a hand, and the gaze lost in the distance.

Another significant moment in the funeral rite and, as I see it, a variant with more primitive characteristics, is the passage from the portrayed gesture, also represented in the figurative and sculptural art of the classical world, to the enacted gesture: for example, the food of the dead in its countless senses.

Depositing food in the sepulchre had the purpose of preventing the hungry dead from coming back among the living to look for it.

This custom is known among the Egyptians but not only there. Its transformative potential can be interpreted both as progressive, given the long arc of time over which it has been maintained, and as regressive because of this transition from symbolic figuration to the absolute concreteness of which we have evidence. In India it was customary to place two shovelfuls of rice or flour in the tomb, while the Persians put a portion of enough food for about three days, after which time they thought the soul would have completely removed itself from the body (De Gubernatis, *Storia dell'etnologia* [History of ethnology], 1912). The Greeks and Romans likewise commemorated their dead with votive offerings of food and wine placed on the tombs, while the Babylonians and Assyrians buried jars of honey.

There is a variety of documentary evidence demonstrating the use of real food in sepulchres in much later times, such as *De Masticatione Mortuorum in Tumulis* (by Michael Ranft,[29] Martini Leipzig, 1728) and the *Dissertatio Historico-Philosophica de Masticatione Mortuorum* by Philip Rohr and Benjamin Fritzsch of 1679, which describe how, if the dead person's food stocks were insufficient, they might nourish themselves by chewing on the shroud and their own flesh.

It is possible to speculate that this conviction originated in experiences of exhumation which revealed the disconcerting outcomes that were probably caused by the tragic consequences of apparently dead people being buried alive. Indeed, we know there were no instruments for establishing the need to wait before burial, and that on the contrary bodies were buried in haste to prevent epidemics. These possible discoveries may have further encouraged the ancient phantasy-myth of the *return of the dead*.

Cannibalism thus became a method for ensuring the deceased's second death, and in fact the stomachs (of the living) would in this way become his or her definitive sepulchre. This interpretation could have given rise to various popular expressions about "drinking" or "eating the dead" (De Martino, 1959), and the custom of the funeral feast is still preserved in Latin America, but also in parts of North America and in the Jewish world. On the Day of the Dead, as if reprising the theme of necrophagy, in communities across Italy sweets in the shape of bones are prepared and called *bones of the dead*.

In fact, cannibalism remains one of the great taboos of Western human thought, as much as or more than incest, and may only emerge as a material act in situations where survival is at stake or in serious psychopathologies. And perhaps for this reason the accusation of cannibalism has been used as a means of propaganda to discredit enemies and opponents. In his book *The Man-Eating Myth: Anthropology and Anthropophagy* (1979) William Arens records the fact that Christians were accused of cannibalism by the Jews, the Irish by the English, the French by the Germans, and vice versa. Peoples who considered themselves civilised consistently accused others of being uncivilised.[30]

From the Palaeolithic era until today, at least three types of cannibalism have been clearly identified.

So-called alimentary cannibalism is practised because of the need for nourishment. Of course this only happens in cases of extreme necessity. It probably occurred among the Neanderthals, the Anasazi, and other Amerindians who introduced the element of cooking, the First People of Australia, and some African nations. There are more recent instances from Russia in the period 1921–1923, during the first famine, and in Ukraine ten years later, in 1931, for the same reason. As recently as 1942, during the Second World War, it was documented that some Russian soldiers had eaten their fellow combatants in Finland.

There are two other forms. *Ritual cannibalism* has been widespread in the past and is still practised today with the magical religious purpose of theophagy. By contrast, in the case of *pseudo-cannibalism* the practices are not literally cannibalistic but are nevertheless connected to the cult of the dead and may leave traces similar to those caused by butchery: for example, stripping the flesh from the bodies of the deceased.

The anguish about the return of the dead has very distant origins which touch on myth and are rooted in it, in particular the myth of Sisyphus. Various versions of the myth exist, one of which tells that Sisyphus had received permission to return to the land of the living, not only from Persephone but from Hades himself, provided that he returned to the land of the dead within one day. In another version of the myth, Sisyphus does not honour the deal made with the divinities of the underworld and stays in the world of the living. It is very likely that from this myth arose the belief that the dead can return, and even feed themselves. With regard to Alcestis, mentioned earlier, it is interesting to recall that when Heracles goes to rescue her and brings her back among the living, he requires her not to speak for three days because she must be decontaminated. We could see this as a sort of deathly consecration which necessitates a rite of passage in order to cross the border, as if signalling the presence of a caesura which is both impassable and pervaded in phantasy by the fear that it may be violated and breached. Feeding oneself on bread prepared in the dead person's home would therefore mean the same as feeding oneself on the deceased themselves, hence the numerous traditions and popular expressions which can be considered a symbolic residue, still present, of these experiences.

But in the ancient world the symbiosis with the dead was also considered a source of regeneration and linked to sexuality, while for Christianity the experience of death is associated with a new hope of rebirth, and the kernel of the grain from which bread is made, which rots in the earth during winter and then bears new fruit, is a recurrent metaphor of resurrection in the Gospels.

So there are interesting funeral traditions with a link to sexuality, of which a trace remained in ritual until even a few decades ago.

The death of a spouse brought to the bereaved family an inevitable *libido deficients*, translated by De Martino (De Martino, 1959) as "*attanassamento*,"[31] a term used in the Lucanian region to indicate a lack that need not, and must not, persist.

This involved an idea of something that in psychoanalysis we know as an increase in the libidinal drive after a death, and it acted with a dual purpose: to reaffirm life, but also to frighten the dead person, almost a warning about the great vital force ranged against them. In any case, obscene display is a way of aggressively manifesting the energy of the living, as Freud also asserts when he recalls that uttering obscenities corresponds to the unleashing of an attack equivalent to a sexual assault, making the listener feel as if they had actually suffered one. So in this case the attack is enacted against the deceased and the purpose is once again apotropaic.

Sexual elements were also present in many cults of the dead in the ancient world. In Egypt the mourners often bared their breasts (De Martino, 1959), ostentatiously displaying a feeling of life and representing the milk that nourishes it.

The transition from the sexual act to laughter, music, and dance corresponds to the search for a more mitigated and less concrete way of expressing aggression. Funeral dances took place in antiquity and these continued as active rituals into the Middle Ages, as is testified by the *Dance Macabre* still present today in many churches and cemeteries.[32]

Mourning in Freud

As I mentioned earlier, Freud was interested in certain anthropological findings which he quotes both in *Totem and Taboo* (1913) and in *Group Psychology and the Analysis of the Ego* (1921). I believe the other anthropological texts I have referred to, and many more, will be helpful in understanding the work that every human being must carry out in relation to loss, which is not only the loss of a single person, since these texts are also proof of the heritage of work on loss carried out by many previous generations who wished to pass this on to the generations who came after them.

This work of mourning, like that of ritual, is a sphere in which there is living testimony in the relationship between the subject and the group.

According to Freud, when the working-through of loss is concluded, the libido previously directed onto the lost object must be transferred onto another object, and an enormous amount of work is also needed to invest in unconscious phantasies and in primal phantasies transmitted transgenerationally.

In fact, in the accounts of rituals, the two axes – vertical and horizontal: the history of the individual and the history of individuals – seem integrated and interwoven in a particularly complex way which demonstrates the synchronicity of several temporal planes: the existential, religious, and historical depicted simultaneously. By using the expression "work of mourning" in *Mourning and Melancholia* (1915a), Freud focuses on the individual and emphasises how this work involves a whole series of conscious and unconscious psychic operations concerned with the affectively and instinctually invested object. When this process is accomplished the subject gradually becomes able to accept the loss and the Ego can once again direct its libidinal investments in another direction.

Before entering the world of Freud's *Mourning and Melancholia* I believe it is necessary to take a step back to *On Narcissism: an Introduction* (1914).

This 1914 work is indeed fundamental, opening the door to the whole Freudian *Metapsychology* (1915) and the two approaches to drive theory, but in my opinion it is also a focal point in the link between the individual and the group.

It does in fact have important repercussions for Freud's conception of the social world because the Ideal of the Ego addressed in the final section of *On Narcissism* becomes a valuable element in addressing a collective and group Ideal of the Ego which is the foundation for great institutions.[33] (This group Ego Ideal still leaves many open questions about social and institutional reality today.)

In mythology, the adventure of Narcissus represents the condemnation of falling in love with one's own image, being incapable of responding to love from the other person. Narcissus rejects Echo's attempts to attract him, but she is punished in turn by the goddess Nemesis, making her speak only the words of others and not her own. Both mythological images seem to represent punishments. Narcissism is a punishment, a nemesis, which in the classical world represented the destined scourge of any tyrannical egocentrism. Narcissus therefore symbolises an authentic structural problem in the Ego's mirroring relationship with itself, and Freud's essay elevates the myth of Narcissus to a metapsychological dimension. So it is not by chance that the *theory of identification* is expounded here, having been posited earlier in *Leonardo da Vinci and a Memory of His Childhood* from 1910, where we find the theoretical bases of the *processes of identification* and of the concepts of *narcissism* and *sublimation.*[34]

Only a year after *On Narcissism*, when Freud was busy with *Mourning and Melancholia* and the narcissistic condition involved in these two psychic realities, he emphasised the possible transformation of the Ego in the relationship with the object. Relations with the primary objects are fundamental to this, enabling the Ego to be well structured and to develop in a way that completes and supersedes the phase of primary narcissism: or conversely, compromising it, which has repercussions for the quality of future object relations. In melancholic disturbance the libido in fact withdraws onto an Ego that in this case is altered or deformed/de-objectified.

Thus, alongside a relation that is characterised by the *desire to have a relationship with the object*, there appears a relation characterised by the *desire for the object to be like an ideal image of the Ego*, resulting in the expectation that the Ego will be mirrored in such a relationship. The frustrations deriving from the disappointments caused by life deviating from the ideal image have an impact on the Ego, which has been incapable of matching up to the ideal expectations. And so a devalued image of the Ego and the object is slowly established in an Ego whose structure has been altered because of problems in moving on to recognition of the object during the phase of primary narcissism. (See also Abraham's developmental studies.) Narcissistic evolution will inevitably have substantial importance for Oedipal evolution, with quantitative and qualitative consequences in later difficulties with separation and relations of dependency.

There is value in recording the inevitable social impact of an individual narcissistic evolution, but it is also good to bear in mind the fact that whole groups can move in this dangerous direction, and Chapter IV will explore these dynamics in more detail.

So, while *narcissism* runs through Freud's entire theory, the question of *mourning*, which entails a specific contribution of narcissism to the process of identification, also inexorably penetrates deeply into these strata.

We know from phenomenology that when faced with an unpleasant impression emerging from the inner or the outside world, the psyche spontaneously strives to get rid of it, casting it into *oblivion*. This means detaching the unpleasure from the representational world in order to inhibit its representations. Indeed, viewed metapsychologically, these representations convey a highly disturbing affect. Once again there is a link to the hypnogenic rituals discussed in previous sections.

Still on a metapsychological level, the representational intensity is bound up with the quantity of psychic energy tied to the recollection. The *work of mourning* uses and, so to speak, consumes the free energy of the affect, committing it to that work and, without altering the sensory image in any way – this being previously employed for the representation – restores it to the subject once the work of mourning is completed, free now from the unbearable affective charge. Note that this must involve taking account of times and quantities which have absolutely individual outcomes and are highly distinct from each other, even when other obstacles do not intervene.

On these factors Freud is clear: mourning needs a certain period of time to be accomplished, during which therapeutic interference is inappropriate and even harmful since, to make the point once again, mourning is a process registered in feelings and not in symptoms unless other elements intrude to alter the picture.

> *Reality-testing* has shown that the loved object no longer exists, and it proceeds to demand that all libido shall be withdrawn from its attachments to that object.... Nevertheless its orders cannot be obeyed at once. They are carried out bit by bit, at great expense of time and cathectic[35] energy, and in the meantime *the existence of the lost object* is psychically prolonged. Each single one of the memories and expectations in which the libido is bound to the object is brought up and hyper-invested, and detachment of the libido is accomplished in respect of it.
>
> (*Mourning and Melancholia*, 1917, pp. 244–245, my italics)

This is how we understand the use of the term *work*, which presupposes a prior activity of bonding since it is a matter of slowly advancing towards an inner detachment with the function of inhibiting the development of melancholia.

Where this bond was absent or deficient, or at least altered, the work of hyper-investment in the image and the subsequent disinvestment in favour of reality-testing is obstructed, becoming difficult, and sometimes even impossible. These are cases of melancholy or complicated mourning. According to Freud, *hyper-investment in the image* and *reality-testing* proceed in parallel.

Which raises the following question: why might a *work of binding* lead to detachment and not to unbinding?[36]

Freud says,

> Each single one of the memories and situations of expectancy which demonstrate the libido's attachment to the lost object is met by the verdict of reality that the object no longer exists; and the ego, confronted as it were with the question whether it shall share this fate, is persuaded by the sum of the narcissistic satisfactions it derives from being alive to sever its attachment to the object that has been abolished.
>
> (*Mourning and Melancholia*, 1917, p. 255)

In the end the object is free, but exhausted by the gradual, wearying labour of disinvestment. We can recognise this not only in the mourning for material losses but also in the difficult analytic and psychotherapeutic task of fostering the work of mourning when it has been deficient or missing from the patient's life, with the aim of "losing" *totalising objects* on which the subject has been strongly dependent (products of sadistic and tyrannical superegoic ways of functioning). These *totalising objects* present themselves in sessions under various guises, personified or otherwise, real and/or ideal, single or multiple, drawn from the subject's present history or present in his or her evolution or life cycle (marriage, the birth of a child, an illness, a problem of infertility, ageing, the menopause, retirement, etc.).[37]

It can be no coincidence that at the same time as he was writing *Mourning and Melancholia*, Freud also wrote *On Transience* (1915), a work in which he describes the tendency to invest minimally in what is beautiful but transient, in order to preserve oneself from an investment that would later compel the subject to suffer for the loss, a suffering that would become intolerable.[38]

This all tells us that the work of mourning has its natural outcome in the separation of the living from the dead so that life can continue to assert itself.

I believe that what happens during the evolution of the human brain moves towards a death that helps the continuing affirmation of life. Indeed, we cannot do without neuronal apoptosis,[39] programmed in early phases of life so that neurons are selected in various ways for the best possible functioning and development, as happens with the branches of a plant after an effective pruning. I would note this too as a representation of the *work of mourning* – work as genetically programmed apoptosis – under the aegis of *Eros*.

By contrast, the refusal to mourn, its accelerated, anticipated development, with little inclination to pass through a grief that has all the dynamic characteristics I have just described, bears the mark of *Thanatos*, the death instinct. Avoiding the process of working-through and gradual disinvestment, it plunges the Ego into an affective void characteristic of the most serious forms of melancholia and its polar opposite, mania.

The persistence of the image in mourning; remembering

If, as Freudian metapsychology records, representation consists of a perceptual quota and an ideational quota which become integrated and compose the thing-representation as well as the word-representation that conveys the represented thing to consciousness, mourning can be considered as an experiential scenario specifically related to the resultant complexity of this difficult integration.

In some pathological situations, but also in others that we could say are more physiological, such as mourning, the bifurcation between idea and perception is widened: the two elements are separated and the image may appear severed from its representation and thus be *presented* instead of *represented*, laden with its now liberated affective component. In fact, Freud points out that during mourning the bereaved subject attempts to prolong the dead person's existence, an attempt that is at odds, though concomitant, with the newly begun work of mourning, and thus characterised by a still dominant ambivalence.

The perceived images of the lost person keep coming back for much longer than any words associated with them, and sometimes almost without any awareness of their persistent presence. They insistently remain like an "occupying power," which keeps them at a distance from possible deformation or representational and ideational re/con-formation, which would be the result of an integration that, it is hoped, would occur in the future.

We may say that what is configured in this case is a tendency to repeat rather than to remember. And we have seen the hypnagocic function of repetitions in funeral rites, a function intended to protect against the grief caused by irreversible separation.

Remembering is a much more congruent and complete experience in which the transitions I mentioned earlier, between imaginative representation and idea, have resumed their flow between unconscious and preconscious which had been deferred until the representative parts were better assembled, and where the quantitative burden is significantly reduced, again thanks to repression. Remembering demarcates the possibility of a passing beyond and being able, in this passing, to fulfil an experience of loss within the psychic system itself.

The *representing of the person who is lost* and subsequently *remembered* is not only a *transformed image*, but is a thoroughgoing process of *deformation* to which the whole psychic apparatus is subjected since the quantity of free affect is reduced because it is being employed in the working-through of mourning.

Repeating, by contrast – in this case linked to the reappearance of the lost person's image – is registered in an initial psychic experience that is opposed to reality and to the need for acknowledgement of the loss on the psychic and experiential level; but at the same time it has the function of distancing the grief, of emptying or discharging part of the free affect that is conveyed with the grief as it re-presents the image that keeps making its reappearance. The inescapable and violent reality of separation is thus filled by the image, cut loose from the idea and from the possibility of thinking it: this is a re-actualisation which is temporarily emptied of sense and developmental potential.

The emptying of sense stands outside consciousness and is in reality a non-sense, as it is regarded *a posteriori* by reactivated thought. (It is a recurrent phenomenon in the observation of mourning by those not directly involved, to wonder why the person left alive is doing things for the dead person that they used to do before, such as ironing their clothes, or performing some surrogate act like going to the cemetery three times a day as a reflection of how many times a day they used to see the lost person.)

In the moment when the image intrudes, the only possible meaning is a celebratory one – ritual: and yet ritual behaviour would appear to be the most suitable kind for accepting and coming to terms with *loss*, since the ritual characteristics of celebration restrain the object and, as Freud says, cause the existence of the lost person to endure.

The celebratory repetition comes to a conclusion alongside the awareness of how this repeating brings a decline in meaning. Thought appears and is retrieved, drawing on the internal perception of the images and connecting to the various reintegrated representational forms aiming at ideation.

When the process comes to a good conclusion it is followed by the definitive abandonment of this image, which could therefore be called a "fill-in image."

I think the sequence of psychic events, which are so exceptional and at the same time recurrent, should be understood not as a once-for-all movement between a before and an after, between one module of functioning and another, but as occurring within a set of functionings where the two modules are co-present, each predominating to varying degrees at different moments in this process and differing in the way they are expressed at distinct times within the same individual, depending on the social and cultural group they belong to.[40]

All of this is unlike from what happens in melancholic loss, where not only does the subject fail to realise what they have lost – and indeed, the object-loss in this case can be regarded as entirely withheld from consciousness – but work on the loss also fails, even though the subject is totally absorbed by it. In fact, it offers no curative reversibility and so can be considered a labour in vain. The "filling-in" in this case is effected by delusion, which instals itself in the crack of incongruity between the high level of self-denigration and the actual (but invisible) justification for it.

In the words of Hamlet, quoted by Freud in *Mourning and Melancholia* (p. 246), "Use every man after his desert, and who shall scape whipping?" (*Hamlet*, Act II scene ii).

Hamlet's words ask us to reflect on the fact that if we adopt a viewpoint that is limited, single, rigid, and fixed – and naturally also ideal – and thus evades reality-testing because of all these features (taking an exaggeratedly dim view of "desert," for example), this will then condition the conclusions reached by the judgement, to the extent that any other outcome is rendered impossible.

In melancholy, Freud observes a primal psychic constellation of "revolt" which is later transformed by developing into melancholic contrition. While the spirit of angry revolt is always more or less present in depressive states and accompanies all manic-depressive defences, as it also does in many borderline states, it is nonetheless true that what remains is merely the impotent rage at not being able to put it into action. This is because the capacity for revolt would entail the Ego having a structure and autonomy which in these cases are defective or have serious gaps, and so rage is the persistent residue of the great fears of failure.

On all the aspects of melancholy and its origins, and likewise its evolutions, I refer to the writings of Freud. In these passages of reflection I have limited myself to looking at the work of disinvesting the image.

The work of mourning renders us capable of taking on the loss and is therefore evidence of an early and successful relationship with the object, since every truly mature object-relationship involves the need and ability to deal with loss. This ability is coupled with evidence of a preserved and always renewable capacity for transformation and movement across bridges (transferential/countertransferential bridges which I referred to at the end of the second chapter, on trauma) and in the not always easy transitions that lead to the encounter with the other: going through a small loss of self in order to re-encounter the other and face new transitions.

The work of mourning also entails a libidinal disinvestment of the lost object through adequate reality-testing, but also an important work on ambivalence towards the object, an ambivalence that is naturally not exclusive to melancholia.

After the overcoming of primary narcissism a trace of it persists in mourning, at a level essential for survival since every form of grief involves the need for a narcissistic withdrawal to tolerate and deal with it, like the need to deal with the resulting ambivalence towards the object arising from a dependency-relationship that is inevitable in this withdrawal.

However, as Freud notes, the love–hate conflict which characterises ambivalence is available to consciousness, so will this proximity make the conflict easier to work through?

Consider these expressions:

"Maramao, why are you dead?"[41]

"And I'm angry with my mother because she left me when I was little."

"It would have been better to separate while we were both alive than to live with the intense love I've experienced and then have the desolation of widowhood."

The second and third statements were made by people in analysis who were still in mourning or had been during their treatment, and who had never been melancholic.

Freud again reminds us that the independent working-through of this ambivalence would be impossible for the melancholic outside the process of analytic treatment since the level of the love–hate conflict is separated from consciousness and pushed far back into the unconscious, and most of the psychic work is directed towards making sure it does not emerge. This makes mourning a complex matter to cope with and stops it being, so to speak, at hand for working through. Obviously something has not gone well before, but it is precisely these slippages that analytic work engages with, dispensing with easy defensive categorisations.

Women in the Bible mourning their fertility

Every case of infertility[42] or problematic fertility prompts mourning[43]: but this may be threatened by the presumption that the human race has a universal right to benefit from its discoveries, and so the mourning sometimes seems impossible to do. Indeed, the frustrating impotence caused by arriving at this limit seems to be overcome by vaulting over it. Then it becomes impossible to dwell in the painful conflict or anguish of loss: instead, denial is used as a defence, and the subject asserts their right to something that in fact principally concerns another subject: the child who is yet to be born.

Here I would like to reread the Biblical stories of women who have seemed to me to act as instruments for opening a dialogue and new questions about mourning, as well as helping us to penetrate further into its complexity.

In *Genesis* we can hear the cry of Rachel to Jacob, "Give me children, or I shall die!" and his reply, "Am I in God's place? It is he who has refused you motherhood" (30: 1, *Jerusalem Bible*). *Genesis* tears open the suffering, melancholic, and angry interiority of a frustration felt as intolerable, unbearable. At the same time Jacob's observation underlines the limits of the human, although we have to say his standpoint is much the easier one. Here it is not only the generic fact of being male but also the cultural fact that in his time polygamy was permitted, making it easy for the man to verify the cause of the couple's infertility, even without modern biotechnologies.

Nevertheless, the culture of the time did provide support for the woman too.

In her great grief, Abraham's wife Sarai, who was able to rely on a greater degree of goodwill than Rachel, turns to Hagar her fertile slave: "Go to my slave-girl. Perhaps I shall get children through her" (*Jerusalem Bible*, 16: 2).

Again in *Genesis*, Rachel too accepts, and even suggests, this solution:

> "Here is my slave-girl, Bilhah. Sleep with her so that she may give birth on my knees [*al birkay*]; through her, then, I too shall have children!".
>
> (*Jerusalem Bible*, 30: 3)

If we look for the meaning of this expression "on my knees" we discover that it is much more profound than its literal translation. The Hebrew term for knees – *birkay* – has the same root as "blessing" (*b-r-kh*) and in the Bible blessing does indeed mean the granting of fecundity and life.

Rachel's action is thus not only a legitimate adoption entitling her to give names to Bilhah's children, but her taking part in the birth becomes a real "cure" for her infertility. Here I want to point out that not only will the children have a name, but that both women name their handmaids and, by naming them, legitimise their role in the event, which is the generation of children and care for the infertile adoptive mothers (Milka Ventura Avanzinelli, *Sterilità e fecondità delle donne bibliche*, 2005, pp. 75–79).

The fates of the two slaves – because they are slaves nonetheless, as the law permitted – will be different: Hagar will flee into the desert because she feels rejected, and her son Ishmael (who lives in Isaac's shadow because of the rivalry between the women) will follow his mother into the desert and be saved there by a compassionate God.

It is true that the pain of Sarai and Rachel still has remarkable historical and cultural significance, but it seems to confirm the oblative quality of a child being *born*, as opposed to being *possessed*. In particular, as Rachel works it through, a gift is offered that can be given and received on several levels, a gift which therefore also plays a part in the working-through of the mourning for not having that gift. It is in fact the working-through of mourning for infertility which enables Rachel to see that in the lack and loss there may also be a gift. It is a gift that is received and given at the same time only in the acknowledgement of an otherness which has contributed to all this, an otherness that always has a name, one that unequivocally marks out every subject. And what is more, Rachel will go on to have children of her own.

Clearly, the pain of infertility is a pain involving mourning which, even as early as the *Book of Genesis*, is indissolubly both psychic and physical.

Another Biblical figure offers evidence of this with even greater intensity in the *First Book of Samuel*. Hannah was Elkanah's favourite wife, but she was infertile. "Hannah, why are you crying?" asks Elkanah. "Why are you not eating anything? Why are you so sad? Am I not more to you than ten sons?" (I *Samuel*, 1: 8). This male, who puts himself almost on the level of a child, seems to a be naïve and hardly responsible means of coping with a desire for parenthood, and yet he has an effect on Hannah's depressive mourning. The moment came when she ate and drank in the temple, and then "got up and stood before Yahweh" (I *Samuel*, 1: 9). (Standing up always indicates the rise of a new life in Biblical and Midrashic texts as well as in the Gospels.) This happens while they are in the temple celebrating the birth of an important child, Obed, ancestor of David and the Messiah.

I am pointing all this out to make clear the context of deep spirituality coupled with deep conflict in this woman: in fact Hannah seems able to store up everything that happens around her, like a sudden rebirth of the subject, but also a laborious but happy rediscovery of the object.

These examples, though so different from each other, nevertheless have one characteristic in common: the deep narcissistic wound caused in the woman by her mourning for infertility. They may be ancient and perhaps forgotten stories, but they are an example of how profound and intense the psychic problem of infertility can be and, regardless of prevailing laws and cultures, how the problem can only be addressed, and perhaps overcome, in a group context. This context begins with the couple and extends to the societal level where the presence and complementarity of the other are sustained by a profound subjective and identitary meaning, but also by the sense of the limit which, added to the spiritual meaning of the Biblical text, finds further opportunities for expression and justification in social recognition by the group. This all has an enormously subjectivating effect: every woman has her own way of making her case; all women have their own path to follow. And the role of the group presence in the mourning for infertility relates back to what I noted at the start of the chapter: the function of ritual to involve groups and sometimes the entire collective, and to be both evidence of support and an instrument for working-through.

All of which challenges the present time's collective, social, and group capacity for dealing with mourning and sustaining its necessary representational role, and brings to our attention more and more frequently the infinite number of ways in which the idea of society is being negated.[44,45]

Poetry, however, keeps its memory alive:

> And white-armed Andromache led their songs of sorrow
> cradling the head of Hector, man-killing Hector
> gently in her arms: "O my husband
> cut off from life so young! You leave me a widow,
> lost in the royal halls – and the boy only a baby,
> the son we bore together, you and I so doomed.
> I cannot think he will ever come to manhood.
> Long before that the city will be sacked,
> plundered top to bottom! Because you are dead,
> her great guardian, you who always defended Troy,
> who kept her loyal wives and helpless children safe…
>
> *Iliad*, XXIV, 718–725

Notes

1 See the studies of structural language by the semiologist Ferdinand de Saussure, picked up by Lacan in relation to the unconscious as structured like a language (*Ecrits*, 1974) and André Green's critique of Lacan's theoretical approach to this (*On Private Madness*, 1986. "Note sui processi terziari" in *Propedeutica: Metapsicologia rivisitata*, 1993).

2 Many of Freud's works, beside those cited, consider the relationship between individual and group, the relationship between the functioning of agencies such as the Superego and social relations, and also the role of spirituality in group identities. I mention these works later, in the first note to the section "Mourning in Freud" in this chapter. In the present note, however, I shall mention *Group Psychology and the Analysis of the*

Ego (1921), *The Ego and the Id* (1923), *The Future of an Illusion* (1927), *Civilisation and Its Discontents* (1929), and *Moses and Monotheism* (1939), written shortly before his death and from a position somewhat detached from *The Future of an Illusion.* I decided to mention these in a note so that readers can explore them further if they wish, preferring not to clutter the text with this vast body of bibliographical material about Freud's oeuvre, in favour of the path I am pursuing in this chapter.

3 In *Gruppo e funzione analitica*, Koinos, 1, pp. 20–27, 2000.

4 Raimon Panikkar Alemany, Spanish philosopher, theologian, priest, and writer, was a twentieth-century spiritual guide and witness to intercultural dialogue and the encounter between religions.
Brunetto Salvarani is a theologian, essayist, and literary critic.

5 Paolo Brezzi: "Il carattere e il significato della storia nel pensiero di Sant'Agostino" [The character and meaning of history in St Augustine's thought] in *Analisi e interpretazione di De Civitate Dei di Sant'Agostino*, pp. 159–163, 1960.

6 Morrou H.-J. *L'ambivalance tu temps de l'histoire chez Saint Augustin*, Conférence Albert Le Grand, Paris 1950. Quoted in Brezzi (1960).

7 For all the distinctiveness of his thinking, St Thomas Aquinas (1225–1274) sees the movement of human consciousness similarly stretching from the immanent universe to the transcendent, and sees that this span is moved by man's own bodily reality, since it was created by God, the first of all movements (Ruffini F. on Aquinas in *La "Quaestio disputata de unione verbi Incarnati"*, 2017). The passing of several centuries brings us to Gian Battista Vico, in whose thought the question of individual history and an ideal, eternal universal history is not solved, but impels us onto a new horizon. In *Scienza Nuova* (Gian Battista Vico, "Principi di Scienza Nuova" in *Opere*, ed. Battistini A., 1990) the philosopher seems able to imagine a mosaic structure, in which the meaning of each element can only be understood in connection with the neighbouring elements. The concept of an eternal, ideal history can only be understood within a contiguous idea, which is that of the history of single nations, expressing the desire for a science capable of adapting itself to the concreteness of existence. This desire becomes a focal point of his thought, which is very remote from that of the early Christian world and the Middle Ages. The well-known courses and recursions of history are offered and interpreted by Vico not as repetitions but as movement in an ascending spiral.

8 The notion of *divine revelation* was also implicit in other religions, but happened in a mythic time and was invoked by the rituals of repetition.

9 I invite my psychoanalyst readers to reflect on the enormous number of dreams by patients during the lockdowns of Covid-19, and likewise the immense quantity of vignettes, jokes, and *jeux d'esprit* recurring on the social networks during the same period, representing a desire for escape, freedom; and also how the dreams testified to persistent psychic activity when everything was grinding to a halt. In the years since, however, the signs of escape have been very different, coalescing into subversive groups and general rebellion. Though this is often interpreted as intolerance of constriction, I believe it can be read as an intolerance of frustration, of having to do without, an inability to mourn, a phobia which has often slipped from avoidance into denial and negation, in extreme cases becoming omnipotence and reality-splitting, justifying rebellion with the use of entirely delusional contents.

10 "The true *cogito* does not define the existence of the subject through the thought the subject has of existing, does not convert the certainty of the world into a certainty of the thought about the world, and finally, does not replace the world itself with the signification 'world.' Rather, it recognises my thought as an inalienable fact and it eliminates all forms of idealism by revealing me as 'being in the world'." (Merleau-Ponty, 1945, *Phenomenology of Perception*, p. lxxvii, 1962). I quote this in support of Merleau-Ponty's concepts of the modes in which being appears to the consciousness of existing and the recursive construction of a new object.

11 Ernesto De Martino (1961), *La terra del rimorso. Contributo a una storia religiosa del Sud* [The land of remorse: contribution to a religious history of the South], 2015. The book is the result of research carried out by De Martino and his multidisciplinary team in Puglia, and in particular the Salento of the 1950s. The research aims to tell the story of a culturally conditioned symbol in a circumscribed geographical area and a clearly defined chronology.

I had known this text for some time and yet it has stimulated my interest again. The link to psychoanalytic thinking hinges on parallelisms and analogies with obsessional rituals, but also on all the clinical situations where repetition dominates, and above all those that are traumatic. Tarantulism found itself strongly opposed by Christianity, probably because of its association with a musical catharsis, the roots of which lie in the orgiastic and initiatory rites of paganism. However, it was also sharply at odds with the new science which rejected what was then considered a magical ceremony. Thus both its rise and its decline remain linked to important moments in the inner history of Western civilisation, and especially that of the geographical area studied by De Martino.

12 Théodore Géricault, *The Raft of the Medusa*, oil on canvas, 1818–1819, Musée du Louvre, Paris.
https://commons.wikimedia.org/wiki/File:JEAN_LOUIS_TH%C3%89ODORE_G%C3%89RICAULT_-_La_Balsa_de_la_Medusa_(Museo_del_Louvre,_1818-19).jpg#/media/File:JEAN_LOUIS_THÉODORE_GÉRICAULT_-_La_Balsa_de_la_Medusa_(Museo_del_Louvre,_1818-19).jpg
The frigate Medusa had left France in 1816 bound for Senegal – a British colony recently ceded to France at the Treaty of Paris – accompanied by three other ships, as was usual on long voyages, but commanded by a relatively inexperienced captain. Thinking to save time and effort, the captain ordered the ship to sail at full speed, causing it to end up on a sandbank. The people left on board without lifeboats built a remarkably large raft – 20m x 7m – but its size made it too heavy and the ropes holding it together soon broke.
Nevertheless, the raft did its job… and it cannot be ruled out that the survivors may have lived thanks to cannibalism, a subject which will return later in this chapter.

13 The *Taranta* is a ritual celebration involving a dance similar to the Tarantella, which derives from it. Taranta is also used to indicate the arachnids, the spiders themselves.

14 Salento is a peninsular region in Puglia, southern Italy.

15 [Translator's note: older forms of English preserved the concreteness of this idea in the Anglo-Saxon "again-bite" (*ayenbite*) of conscience, a link obscured by the exclusive use of the Latin term "remorse" in modern English.]

16 My italics. I wanted to emphasise the efficacy and precision of the term used by De Martino. This is not a matter of *representation*, the result of a good integration between perception and ideational elements related to it and to reality-testing. What is proposed here is a *figuration*, from the Latin *fingere*, understood in the sense of "insisting," "bending." It is an insistence on the configured object, aiming – indeed striving – towards representing it. See, inevitably, *La figurabilité psychique* by César and Sara Botella.

17 See Chapter II.

18 The relationship between Otto Rank and Freud has been controversial. Rank was a highly cultivated Viennese philosopher and intellectual who, though he had not been analysed, was instantly admitted by

Freud into the Wednesday Society where he took the minutes. He also became a member and Secretary of the International Psychoanalytic Association and editor of *Imago* – Journal for the Application of Psychoanalysis to the Sciences of the Spirit – the first psychoanalytic journal, founded in 1912a. He was highly regarded by Freud who felt a deep friendship for him, as was also demonstrated by the fact that Rank's papers *Dream and Poetry* (1914) and *Dream and Myth* (1914) were cited in the appendix to chapter 6 of *The Interpretation of Dreams*, from the fourth to the seventh editions (i.e., from 1914 to 1930). In *Mourning and Melancholia* Freud also took up some of Rank's observations on the aspects of narcissism involved in melancholia. In fact it is still uncertain whether the very term narcissism had been coined by Freud or transcribed, as a summary of a Freudian thought, by Rank in the Wednesday minutes, and thus first coined by him. Again, in *The Uncanny* (1919) Freud turned to some of Rank's theories, in particular the *theory of the double*. Later, in 1923, Rank and Sándor Ferenczi wrote an innovative paper on *The Development of Psychoanalysis* (published in 1924) where "repeating" is preferred to "remembering" and what is considered a passive analytic listening is challenged by a new technique said to be "active." Here, however, real problems began to arise for Freud, partly because he had absolutely no inclination to practice this active technique, at least as the two authors were proposing it, but above all because he was wholly at odds with them over the question of how long treatment should last. Many years later, in *Analysis Terminable and Interminable* (1937a), Freud makes his position clear on this, standing against any defined time period for analysis, opposing any offer of brief therapies or even the setting of a fixed term to analysis. We cannot overlook the fact that by 1937 Freud was in his eighties and had undergone very painful therapy on his cancer of the jaw, so it is difficult, and in any case makes little sense, to interpret Freud's decision about timing in relation to these other propositions. Nevertheless, historians have not situated the break between Freud and Rank in this question or this date, but have mostly attributed it to the theory propounded by Otto Rank in his principal work on birth trauma *Das Trauma der Geburt* (1924), which shifted the focus of observation away from the theory of the Oedipus complex. Later authors have credited Rank with exactly this, that he foregrounded the mother's fundamental and pre-Oedipal role in the relationship with the child at the expense of the later Oedipal relationship with the father. For this reason, many analysts after him – for example, H. Hartmann, W.E.D. Fairbairn, D. Winnicott, H. Kohut, O.F. Kerber, and M. Mahler, as well as Melanie Klein – are directly or indirectly considered his successors. It should be added that the line of thought about the importance of the mother–child relationship was also dear to Jung – *Symbols and Transformations of the Libido* (1912b) – and the fact that it was privileged over the Oedipus complex was one of the decisive factors in the split between Jung and Freud. Moreover, from 1924 to 1926, perhaps also in response to the birth trauma theorised by Rank, Freud reformulated the theory of anxiety, only introducing the concept of ego-splitting in his last works. On the splitting of the ego, I refer again to Otto Rank's important contribution on the *theory of the double* cited by Freud in *The Uncanny* (1919). Rank also later reformulated some concepts of Nietzsche and Jung, re-adapting the concept of the archetype, describing an ego-forming process carried out by the Self, thinking in terms of a creative energy that works in favour of the principle of individuation, and giving weight to the idea of the collective. In 1934, after constant shuttling between Europe and America, he settled in New York and associated with artists and intellectuals impressed by his theory of art: among them, Henry Miller and Anaïs Nin.

19 In *On Narcissism: an Introduction* Freud in fact returns to this perspective, identifying two modes of object-choice: a narcissistic type and an "attachment" type. In melancholia, object-investment is weak because the Ego is structurally weak from the outset: this is Otto Rank's idea, which Freud takes up and endorses. The object-choice has been made on a narcissistic basis earlier in development, and so object-investment may regress to narcissism if difficulties are encountered later in life. This characteristic, a feature of depression, is not predetermined in mourning. According to Freud, this is what enables mourning to have developmental possibilities which in most cases are positive.

20 Karl Abraham was a German doctor who died very young, at the age of forty-seven, much loved by Freud, who called him "my rock of bronze." He tried to urge psychoanalysis towards a study of the psychoses, which was done later under a different theoretical profile by one of his analysands, Melanie Klein. To this end he founded the Psychoanalytic Polyclinic in Berlin and his research was directed above all to the earliest, pregenital developmental stages of the libido, in order to identify the psychosexual differences between schizophrenia and hysteria. With these studies of the developmental history of the libido, he shed light on some points of continuity between hysteria and

psychosis, describing an excess of object-investment in hysteria, a principal cause of ambivalence, while in schizophrenia he found the loss of both object-love and of sublimation, with a consequent regression to autoerotism. He was President of the International Psychoanalytical Association. With Hanns Sachs he convinced Freud to participate indirectly, despite his great puzzlement, in the making of the film *The Mysteries of a Soul (Geheimnisse einer Seele)* of 1926 directed by Georg Wilhelm Pabst which, as well as having great success, contributed to the dissemination of Freudian thought. The surrealists took up psychoanalytic ideas with great enthusiasm, and who can say if the film might also have encouraged the awarding of the Goethe Prize to Freud.

21 I find it noteworthy that the entry on *persistent and complicated mourning* has only recently been added to DSM-5.

22 [Translator's note: Lucania was a region of Southern Italy corresponding to the modern Basilicata.]

23 Book of the Dead of Hori, c.1969–945 BC (papyrus): www.meisterdrucke.it/kunstwerke/1260px/Egyptian_21st_Dynasty_-_Book_of_the_Dead_of_Hori_c1969-945_BC_%28papyrus%29_-_%28MeisterDrucke-916833%29.jpg
In this figure the mourner's "gesture" would seem intended as a form of protection for the deceased: one arm is raised towards his head while the other stretches forwards with the palm upturned, a gesture which has subsequently assumed a protective character rather than one of defence.

24 The Rite of Beating used to take place in the province of Benevento, at Guardia Sanframondi, and regularly formed part of the Feast of the Assumption in mid-August. The fifteenth-century legend tells of oxen kneeling before a statue of the Madonna which emerged from the earth and became immoveable. The peasants were convinced that a general penance was necessary and began to flagellate themselves according to the Mediaeval ritual. Then it became possible to move the statue, which was believed to have become lighter because of the penance. From that date onwards, a week-long procession was held every seven years to expiate the sins of the community.

25 For the ancient world, and especially for the Greeks, not only mimicry but the whole body is an expression of the world. The gesture and the movements of the body which accompany it express an inner state of mind. The *schemata* thus summarise the forms of these gestures.

26 See the *prothêsis* scene, detail of a *krater* from around 715 BCE, Musée du Louvre: https://commons.wikimedia.org/wiki/File:Prothesis_Dipylon_Painter_Louvre_A517.jpg#file

27 Sarcophagus of Tanagra, Minoan period, c.1200 BCE. One iconographic analysis speculates that the figures drawn on this sarcophagus are not women, as on almost all the other *larnakes*, but men. The hypothesis is based on the fact that they are wearing caps used in sacred rites to which only men were admitted. This would also be confirmation that men did indeed take part in funeral rites usually performed by women: https://dynamic-media-cdn.tripadvisor.com/media/photo-o/17/8c/0c/b3/larnax-sarcofago-del.jpg?w=1400&h=-1&s=1

28 *Loutrophòros* is a vase that was used for the water of purification in sacred rituals to wash women before their wedding and the bodies of unmarried women who died young; the vase was then left in the tomb. In Jewish funeral rites the purification of the corpse by liberal application of running water or through immersion in a bath is still a ritual for preparing the corpse – *Taharah* – which is completed with the rite of *Kaddish* for the burial.

29 Michael Ranft, an eighteenth-century Lutheran pastor and expert on vampires, author of *Diceria del vampiro. De masticatione Mortuorum in tumulis* [Rumour of the vampire: on chewing by the dead in burial mounds], 1728.

30 Arens deals with the propagandising use made of this taboo to discredit others in times and places more or less distant from us. Nevertheless, we can establish that this mode of behaviour is less exceptional than may be supposed. It may be used not only to cast a slur on other people by accusing them of being cannibals but also widely used as a metaphor. When a certain group of people chooses to name themselves after a fish and their adversary displays a cat or a dolphin are they not exploiting this atavistic model in metaphorical form? And would this not have been equally threatening or discrediting? We can speculate that the message would have been well received by the fish people who responded in another context by displaying the usual fish, but hugely enlarged, and inviting the adversary to try and eat it. All terribly current, at least until a little while ago when it was Covid-19 that was trying to eat us humans.

31 A portmanteau term in the local dialect combining *Thanatos* (death) and torture with pincers (*tenaglia*).

32 See: Peter Brueghel the Elder, *The Triumph of Death*, 1562, Prado Museum. https://upload.wikimedia.org/wikipedia/commons/1/10/Thetriumphofdeath.jpg
Unknown artist, *The Triumph of Death*, fifteenth-century fresco, 600 × 642 cm, Palazzo Abatellis (Palermo), currently in the Galleria Regionale della Sicilia (Palermo). The date of the painting is unknown like that of its artist, but it is known that the work was commissioned around 1400: www.museoradio3.rai.it/dl/portali/site/articolo/ContentItem-9ac80807-faf0-4145-9589-ed1704753820.html
See also: Buonamico di Martino, known as Buffalmacco: 1336–1341, fresco 560 cm × 1,500 cm, Campo Santo Monumentale, Pisa: https://upload.wikimedia.org/wikipedia/commons/8/84/Buonamico_Buffalmacco_001.jpg
Finally: Dance of Death, Oratorio dei Disciplinati, Clusone, Bergamo: https://cosedibergamo.com/2019/12/31/4-curiosita-su-la-danza-macabra-e-il-trionfo-della-morte-di-clusone/

33 This fundamental work from 1914 will not be developed further on Freud's theoretical journey. Nevertheless there is still an echo of it under the radar in many of his works, always with regard to this relationship between the Ideal of the Ego and the group. Note *Group Psychology and the Analysis of the Ego* (1921) which highlights the instinctual impulses with special attention to the relationship between the individual and mass society, the heritage of tradition and historical continuity. See also *The Ego and the Id* (1923) where the identification of the psychic agencies is the theme of the whole work and the Superego restores a transgenerational tie. See *Civilisation and Its Discontents* (1929), which corresponds closely to what is addressed in this chapter since prohibition, privation, and frustration are the phases through which the Superego imposes a renunciation of the drives, which are understood as a threat of the re-emergence of the greatest taboos: incest and cannibalism. See *Moses and Monotheism* (1938), written shortly before his death: here, from a viewpoint at odds with *The Future of an Illusion* (1927), he sees spirituality as an instrument of withdrawal from witchcraft, an individual and group practice, and at the same time a helpful challenge to the risk of excessive sensoriality.

34 Leonardo recalls that while he was in his cradle a kite had opened his mouth with its tail (symbolic representation of *fellatio*). The translation was challenged by Shapiro as referring instead to a vulture, and later challenged again by Eissler. But Freud commented that the initial critiques were irrelevant to the idea being expressed in the text.

Freud saw Leonardo as feeling a narcissistic love for himself, being *identified* with young men like himself, and at the same time trying to love himself through identification with the loveable mother. From this, Freud also draws out the idea of *sublimation*: the strong infantile curiosity about sexuality, coming too early and being equally quickly and intensely repressed, leaves a residue in the subject as curiosity and a true epistemophilic passion for study and investigation. Hence, Freud stresses the passage from erotic inhibition to an eroticisation of thought which is typical of sublimation, and of which Leonardo is a matchless example.

35 [Translator's note: although Strachey's "cathectic" and "cathexis" are retained in the *Revised Standard Edition*, they appear less and less often in anglophone psychoanalytic writing. Except in this quotation from Freud, throughout the present book I have preferred to reflect the fact that the standard rendering of Freud's *Besetzung* in Italian (and French) psychoanalytic writing is "investment."]

36 I stress the difference between *detachment* and *unbinding*. On this, see Freud's drive theory and the work of overcoming primary narcissism. Unlike libidinal unbinding, typical of the psychoses and all pathologies founded on the defensive systems of splitting and its derivatives, and where the unbound energy flows into the death instinct, the libidinal energy in mourning concludes an investment and is shifted onto another object: it is bound, unbound, and re-bound. For greater precision, see also André Green. In his representation of the libidinal ties, the concept of *liaison–déliaison–reliaison* indicates an unbinding for the purpose of rebinding – unbinding as part of a transitory investment – as distinct from unbinding as a progressive and definitive goal, which corresponds instead to the death instinct.

37 And perhaps, outside clinical work, our collective and social experience of the Covid pandemic insistently posed us this question about how far the collective is capable of mourning with its usual habits and its narcissistic needs when faced with such a pervasive and destructive reality, at group, societal, and institutional levels.

38 As an illustration of *totalising objects* I refer the reader to the enormous increase in plastic surgery, the extensive use of sildenafil citrate – better known as Viagra – and aesthetic transplants and prostheses. However, before seeing these tendencies as pathological variants, they must be considered in relation to the limitations or differences imposed by social and cultural differences on them. The saying "Better one day as a lion than a hundred as a sheep" would not give the lie to this

tendency. And so we should not forget the reaction formations which run in parallel to repression.

39 *Apoptosis*: intracellular genetic programming of cellular death, present in every cell of the human body (Kerr et al., 1972). In the neurones in particular, there are early phases of *apoptosis*, also programmed, aimed at improving the set-up of each individual's neuronal provision. Forms of *Autism* are characterised by the lack of these early phases of *apoptosis*, resulting in neuronal overcrowding and a range of synaptic complications.

40 This is another reason for taking a long-term view of the consequences of the enormous losses caused by Covid-19 across the world. At the end of May 2020, in a Latin American nation, deaths were being recorded at the rate of one every minute. Nevertheless, beyond the enormous scale of the loss, the process of mourning as I have described it so far was aggravated by the social distancing imposed on relatives who could not be with the dying or see the dead, or even participate in their funeral rites, because lockdowns prevented it. Abruptness and acceleration – naturally justified as safeguarding everyone against infection – certainly did not foster the gradual process of separation that is required for a good outcome of mourning.

41 A jaunty mock lament for the death of a cat which became a popular song in 1939 and was promptly banned by Mussolini for apparently satirising the death of the senior Fascist Galeazzo Ciano. The words had appeared in print in 1928 at a time when grief for the mass deaths of the First World War was still acute.

42 What happens to a child born in the age of the biotechnologies? This is the question asked by Paola Marion in the second part ("Being born in the age of biotechnology") of her book *Sexuality and Procreation in the Age of Biotechnology* (2017). The author reverses the view of desire, foregrounding that of the newborn or the baby about to be born, and prioritising the child's desire over the parents'. Marion investigates the child to understand what kind of desire led to its birth – and indeed if its birth was the result of a desire – and the more or less distressing influence that all of this may have on the child's destiny. The book is of great interest for its wide-ranging and proleptic content and its reminder of Piera Aulagnier's question "desire for the child or desire of the child?" but it also prompted me to reread the stories of several women in the Bible – some of them cited in Marion's book – and to use these as models for probing more deeply into the mourning for infertility.

43 We should honestly remind ourselves that every case of infertility, and likewise all fertility, is marked by mourning, although the lost objects are different: in the first case the potential for conceiving and in the second the period of life that was free from the responsibilities which accompany all of parenthood. (In this context, we note the substrate of potential perinatal psychoses.)

44 For the innumerable ways in which society is negated, see Roberto Esposito's book *Politica e negazione. Per una filosofia affermativa* [Politics and negation: towards an affirmative philosophy], 2018.

45 As a reference to more recent times, the inordinate number of deaths from Covid-19 initially brought together two modes of collective behaviour, often with no integration between them. On the one hand there was great fear, so people glued themselves to the television as if every journalist or entertainer were expected to find the right person, the *Deus ex machina* who would give the right, reassuring, definitive answer. On the other hand there was a particular kind of waiting, full of expectations, for the government's evening press conference, which was in fact a bulletin from a war zone. Surprisingly, many patients in analysis reported feeling almost relieved by these, but behind the supposed reality-testing, there was not infrequently a sort of subterranean but still apparent *Schadenfreude*: in the Hebrew expression *simcha-la-ed*, which could be translated as "gladness that it hasn't affected me." While this is a long way from sadism, it is also a long way from possible working-through of mourning, and even from being perceived by consciousness, as is quite frequently the case in massive collective traumas.

IV

PRESENT AND CURRENT/ACTUAL

Multiple and heterogenous identity – identity denied

The human movements which have peaked in the full-scale migrations of this past decade have often had interconnected causes such as climate change, wars, poverty, and the reactions of those who have received the migrants or witnessed them passing through.

As is very well-known, we are currently living at a critical crossroads between the traumatic effects of climatic and environmental change and the equally extreme and traumatic consequences for the possibility of survival where nature is dying. Drought, poverty, and tyranny cause frequent mass migration, bringing political and economic problems to Western societies and having traumatic effects on the life experience, and the very identity, of individuals forced to migrate. They have to engage with a new continent and the customs of new people who are rarely welcoming, while at the same time facing every imaginable kind of difficulty as they try to survive and maintain their human dignity in a manner coherent with their origin and yet open to the rules, laws, and habits of the host country. On the other hand, the people of the host country have the complex and sometimes difficult role of living with the new arrivals, not treating them like intruders, enemies, and thieves and fighting them, but working to *recognise* the different unknown inside each person. At this time there seems to be much work in progress to resolve identitary traumas on the individual and collective levels.

This inevitably leads the psychoanalytic community to reflect on the consequences for identity which accompany these phenomena.

 DOI: 10.4324/9781003747581-5

So these events become an opportunity for a psychoanalytic rethink about the multiple and heterogenous features involved in an identitary structure, and the psyche's complex, controversial systems of denial as they engage with collective and societal reality.

My aim in this is to highlight a structural temporality in these events and to highlight how this may be attacked and transformed by the impact of traumatic events which involve both the collective and the individual to a significant extent, as can be revealed in analytic treatment.[1]

I will try to explore this topic using a specific identity of my own, that of a psychoanalyst, but also with the sense of belonging to a wider identity which, without losing any of my own identity's specific features, can be interlinked with other disciplines in the same spirit that characterises the other chapters.

From a literary perspective, the academic and scholar Arrigo Stara also wrote about the importance of encountering a range of disciplines:

> Whether we think of Leonardo's personality as studied by Freud, or the personalities of characters in fiction… they all clearly had "an identical psychic structure" founded on invasiveness, on the insuperability of "primary narcissism": examples include those of Hoffmann, von Chamisso, Poe, Dostoevsky, Stevenson, Wilde and many others…. That complex and still obscure force [of the psychic structure] seems to need reference to the productions of artistic creativity in order to be explicated… as if literature and art knew it best from having spoken about it first, and with knowledge of its cause.[2]
>
> ("Dell'insolenza dell'io. *Homo Fictus* nella cultura del narcisismo" [On the insolence of the ego: *Homo Fictus* in the culture of narcissism], Breccia (2014), p. 49)

The question of identitary heterogeneity is of particular interest to analysts because the heterogenous character is a fundamental constitutive element of psychic life as a whole, from Freud's concept of drive and representation to the acknowledged valence of the emotions or the more recent understanding of the somatoses. Heterogeneity as a feature absorbed into aspects of the identity may also become an important lens through which to read certain societal phenomena which, although analysts are not always called on to investigate them, cannot be regarded as exempt from the need for a long hard look.

This last reason means that psychoanalysis should take time for reflection on at least two points. First, how much opportunity it has for learning from major historical phenomena such as migration; nationalist identities; the new and multiple sexual identities; identities totally or partly denied in a misogynistic failure to respect the sexual differences between male and female, leading in extreme cases to femicide; and cases of severe narcissistic disturbance, where the inability to tolerate the other's difference creates the desire to possess and control the other, and where this control fails the other's identity must be completely suppressed. Identities are denied in the various forms of exploitative employment; as are the identities of the terminally ill or sufferers from chronic illness who find themselves in a state of almost total dependency on others. But I would not want to forget the denied identities of subjects who were presumably healthy to begin with but defenceless, such as children and young people abused, ignored and downtrodden in various ways that damage their existential complexity.[3]

Second, what psychoanalysis can offer as a contribution to understanding these things. Rather than being solely theoretical – and sometimes defensively so – psychoanalytic understanding should promote reflection – on the collective and group levels too – between the various components in play: political, societal, historiographical, ethical, and cultural.

The term identity is not habitual with Freud: he mentions it in *The Interpretation of Dreams* (1900) in connection with the return of perceptual identity, or names it without dwelling on it at length in some of his references to subjectivity and the composite uniqueness of the individual.

I wonder if this lack of familiarity and this evocation of the *Unheimlich*[4] are the reason for the dismissal of this term "identity," sometimes amounting to an aversion, in a part of modern psychoanalysis. This is an attitude which recurs, though rarely, as the habit of taking a term or concept and completely decontextualising it from a thought that endorses or criticises it, belittling it as a banality, as if a word or statement can be banal in itself, detached from the thought of the person using it, and paradoxically as if this very operation did not risk making the critic's own thought seem banal. It is true that certain concepts are sometimes used "fashionably," so to speak, a use that certainly deserves to be criticised because it is precisely the defensive use or abuse made of them that is not being noticed. Freud puts us on guard against this attitude in the famous note to *Analysis Terminable and Interminable* (1937) when he reminds us about the defensive uses analysts sometimes make of theory, and invites them to undertake periodic analytic treatments (a famous note, and I quoted it earlier, but it is all too often ignored). Obviously the same defensive use can be made of criticism, sending it down the same slippery slope as the person being rebuked. The term "identity" has been, and still is, attacked by one part of psychoanalysis, but of course the term "trauma" has been no better treated, as if the over-simplification lay not in the way a concept is dealt with but in the mere fact of naming it.

The conceptualisation of "identity" was recently addressed in an interesting volume from the French literature which gathers a range of contributions on the *Folies de la norme* (2019). From these, I refer the reader to the chapters by Viviane Abel Prot and André Beetschen which address identity and reflect respectively the two current ways of valuing and devaluing the term identity.[5]

Though identity was not a term used in our sense by Freud, a key concept in Freud is *identification*.

In *Group Psychology and Analysis of the Ego* (1921) he talks about *primary identification* as the most primal form of affective link with the object, which in this phase of development precedes affective investment of the object, an object-investment that will be postulated and articulated in *The Ego and the Id* (1923). The concept of identification thus traces the subject's prehistory and anticipates all the subsequent processes of identification. Primary identification is a direct and immediate kind of identification which, moreover, separates the Id from the Ego-Ideal, leading over time to the conflicts derived from the limitations imposed by a Superego as depository of *secondary identifications* which come to be differentiated during the Oedipus complex.

However, identity was widely discussed well before this in philosophical circles, beginning with Kantian *apperception* which we could transpose, in highly condensed form, onto what Freud attributes to certain structural characteristics of the Ego. The Ego, inevitably immersed in the unconscious because of its penetration into and derivation from the Id, possesses perceptual and synthetising functions which are characteristic of its role as mediator between the three psychic agencies and the outside world, but are also its basis, its constitutional foundation. In the second model Freud goes on to represent perception as having a new valence rather than being a merely reductive product of consciousness; in fact, he considers it as a device for knowing the agencies, and in the *Outline* (1938) he goes so far as to call it a psychic quality.

So a re-reading of the Freudian corpus may lead us to consider identity as a sort of historical memory of the various configurations that the Ego has assumed through perception of the experiences with the objects in which it is identified and the outside world.[6] It is an Ego operating within the single individual and that precise subject in relation to the history that concerns it, *its* history, and thus to all the parental models that have preceded it and lie deposited transgenerationally in its identity-forming experience. These deposits accompany the many early investments deposited in objects. It is thus by virtue of this plasticity of the mind, in continuous and lively motion by means of its re-combinatory capacities, that the features which contribute to the identity are sufficiently multiple and heterogenous, from the archaic residues to the combining and re-combining with experiences deriving from current relationships and the re-actualising of relationships, as in the transference.

This is why both personal and impersonal elements dwell in the identitary experience of every individual, thus rendering it completely heterogenous, a feature to which I will return later in the chapter.[7]

The strongly psychic character of the elements that compose the identity also inevitably renders them open to the unconscious, just as they are founded in it, as we have seen from the first processes of identification, and so they are also necessarily involved in conflictual dynamics correlated both with the urging of desire and with the most primitive defence of unity and integrity/wholeness.

This last feature is significant in traumatic experiences and particularly in experiences of severe and wide-ranging trauma such as genocides, and above all the *Shoah* (on this see Chapter V).

The topic calls for analysts' attention both in clinical practice, recognising it in the narcissistic pathologies and especially in borderline states, and in relation to other disciplines and to society as a whole. I am thinking here about the very substantial forms of splitting that confront us more and more often, and the major current historical significance of certain group phenomena such as those we recognise in religious fundamentalism, terrorism, anti-semitism, xenophobia, and every kind of phobic and expulsive behaviour – which can move from words to deeds – directed at any kind of otherness-difference, with the serious consequences that this is all having on single individuals, groups, and society as a whole.

In the most challenging narcissistic sufferings it is not uncommon for analysts to find themselves having to mirror things that did not happen or that turn out to be impossible to verify one way or the other because what has been experienced and perceived could not be tied symbolically to any representational object.[8] It is therefore impossible to give meaning to an experience which the subject is clinging to like the survivor of a shipwreck. These are extreme situations, always on the edge of catastrophe, where it is sometimes the quantum of *impersonal* identity that seeks an identitary mirroring in the transference-object.

This search is often the expression of an attempt to bring an end to mere survival. Although a secure possibility of life has so far been negated, leaving life hypothecated into the future, survival has nevertheless been the one thing the subject has been capable of guaranteeing and so it is precious because it has left a space open to the potential for becoming. (I will return to the concept of survival, developing it in the chapters that follow. However, I want to stress once more how the search for a guarantee of survival, hypothecating the possibility of life to a date in the future, is a traumatic characteristic which appears in many contexts.)

Even so, historical situations continue to prompt important questions, making the parallels of past and present reverberate with distressing and troubling images such as the tragic experiences of Nazism and all the forms that dictatorship has taken in very recent historical time. These are situations in which personal identity is fused and confused with an extreme, ideological, tyrannical group identity: such an identity is phobic about comparing itself positively with any alterity that has not been turned into a homologue of itself.

These realities are associated with extreme identitary solutions where personal identity – already compromised for various reasons – collapses into an impersonal identity. At this point the two expressions of identity do not confront one another while remaining distinct but are superimposed, making the necessary distinction between them impossible. Their solution is *uniqueness* and *primacy*, which reassure subjects afflicted by the loss of heterogeneity and multiplicity, a loss they are unable to repair. When this happens all potential for change is prohibited (see Chapter VI).

Among the authors who have addressed these phenomena in their psychosocial aspect as well as psychoanalytically, I would like to mention René Kaës (*Le Malêtre*, 2012) and the psychoanalyst and philosopher Cornelius Castoriadis, and to whom I will return on the subject of great traumas like genocide (Chapter V). In some of his reflections, also cited by Kaës in *Le Malêtre*, he emphasises the extent to which, in the transmission of processes of identification, *the contradiction between individualism and conformism*, both so dominant in contemporary society, is *only apparent*. Conformism is possible when a sufficiently important and solid nucleus of identity is diminished or weakened. Then a fictitious nucleus of identity is founded on conformism, based on acritical consensus, magmatic fusion, a sort of collage of multiple identifications to which individualism is allied as in a reaction-formation.

Some aspects of these identities could be described as *unglued*, lacking an integrative experience and the possibility of being represented. They are also noted by René Roussillon (Chapter V), who interprets them as a substitute for the processes of symbolisation. The substitution of a non-symbolic bond in place of the symbolic bond would thus leave a trace of unverifiability about the trauma that has happened, and even about the experience of reality.

It becomes clear just how often the two aspects, individualism and conformism, coexist in some current group expressions. While I am fully aware that Jihadist terrorism is a highly complex and mutable phenomenon where all simplification is very dangerous, nevertheless I want to highlight the way the two aspects function in its destructive attacks, sustained by certain xenophobic and misogynistic tendencies which are given a voice by this form of terrorism – like other mass movements that are only apparently less destructive.[9] Individualism and conformism, far from being mutually contradictory, actually work side by side and support each other in a sort of splitting at such a high quantitative level that it overwhelms any interpretative logic or possible criticism. We must resist any movement along that ideological path, which sustains the splitting and indeed becomes part of it.

Many examples from art, history, and literature,[10] along with others from history and the present day, have shown us how expulsion may be caused by a desubjectivating mechanism for denying identity.

The genocides of history, and massacres generally as part of warfare, like the everyday phenomenon of domestic homicides aimed at suppressing the other – usually a woman who will no longer submit to abuse – show that this oppression, even if it claims to be in defence of an identity, is in fact a refusal to recognise either heterogeneity or the identity-forming processes of those other people, and it goes to extreme lengths to deny their subjectivity.

The paradoxical character of these expulsive phenomena lies in the fact that the denial of the other's identity is imposed in defence of another identity which is opposed to it: for example, the couple, the family, or a supposed role arbitrarily attributed to a person, an ethnic group or a nation, and their supposed primacy, precisely because the first element to be denied is heterogenous identity.

Moreover, identity as the heritage of every subject's individual growth within their own distinctive community can never be a mere possession.

Sometimes homicides are psychic, as in paedophilia and the sexual abuse of minors generally, which often occurs in the family, but for the perpetrator, even in these cases, a supposed possession of the other seems in a completely diseased manner to justify the negation of the victim's otherness and identity. And let us not forget that another form of oppression, quite different in kind, can be imposed on children by those who use them for promotional purposes with no respect for their privacy. As analysts we know that the idea of possession prompts us to investigate a spectrum of defences which are still quite primitive in maturational terms and resort to omnipotence in order to exert desubjectivating control over the other: but possession also suggests many other lines of enquiry. These include the question about whether pathological defences interact, mutually reinforcing each other like phobias and denial, and phobias leading to denial. So perhaps femicides are not so different, in the archaic movements which provoke them, from "homocides" (*Omocidi*, Pini, 2002). The fear of the other, onto whom the power of annulment is projected, could arise from a common projective fear that one's virility, understood as primacy of the male identity, may be compromised or called into question. Could the expansion and radicalisation of all this lead such an individual to take extreme measures and suppress the object of his projection? The deviation of the drives involved in this short-circuit into less highly developed defensive systems associated with the need for identitary primacy may first bypass and then reverse castration (see *Destins de l'autoérotisme*, Chervet et al., 2018).

If respect for privacy is to be more than lip service or a mere legal device, and is to respect the subjectivity of that individual, especially a minor, it is not enough to pixelate or blur the image, or issue a disclaimer. There must be a mode of communication that keeps the child safe from further traumas. Support for this or that opinion about the event is usually not politically neutral, or neutral about the use made of the child and about the child – for example, to seek crowd-funding for a child's expensive medical treatment, all in the name of so-called "free expression." Much is still lacking in this more complex aspect of child protection, both legislatively and culturally: while guaranteeing a due freedom of information, the channels of communication need better regulation, including rules that are more respectful of these young, emergent subjectivities we read about in news bulletins, documentaries, and the kinds of publicity I have just mentioned.[11]

In the same way, the complex questions of trans-identity are often resolved in a brutal manner – whether sex-change treatment is offered or denied – with a failure to listen to the many biological, genetic, historical, and psychic complexities of each individual case. Meanwhile homophobia is on the increase, together with other expulsive phobias about groups outside the dominant one. Perhaps it would be better to say, where there is a dominant group, that is, when a representative democracy is called into question, that those who align themselves with this subversive impulse aim to exclude, and ultimately eliminate, every otherness that does not fit with their position.

Moving onto psychoanalytic ground, we can try to translate the host of situations that have an impact on today's historical reality. A good narcissistic dialectic between self and other which, in a healthy enough functioning, should be formed during development, may in psychoanalytic treatment add substance to the reality-testing that has already happened with the object-Ego and may strengthen the sense of continuity with other objects.

Narcissism is a physiological phase of development and, as such, is fundamental and structural, just as it is fundamental to separate oneself from it in order to encounter the other; but this fruitful encounter with an object other-than-self will never happen successfully if there has not been an initiating encounter with the subject's own Ego seen as separate from the self: in other words, as an object.

And so the dialectic between the feeling of a personal identity and that of an impersonal identity – an obscure and disturbing feeling, in some ways *unheimlich* – is as difficult and complex as it is indispensable, fundamental for existential development, and important for any theoretical approach.

Indeed, theoretical thinking is never without conflict because it is designed by its nature to be compared with other thinking, and potentially refuted. The question is therefore where we situate the conflict and where we situate ourselves with regard to it: but how far is it really possible for us as analysts to put ourselves to one side when we take on our patients' lateral transferences as a complement to our work on the countertransference? More broadly, and thinking beyond psychoanalysis, how possible is it to set ourselves aside when taking on the other-than-us? And yet, picking up the narcissistic dialectic in the individual is very different from making it start in an extended group, which by its very nature avoids the chance of, and wish for, a cure.

However, it may become a real investment that is sometimes coloured by the sacredness of hope. It seems to me that psychoanalysts, in their secular thinking, should pay attention to this good investment in the future and in leaving a legacy, which entails separation, and therefore loss and mourning, so that treatment can include a historicising re-signification of the past. This re-signification is essential for its guarantees to the future; what is kept safe by this safekeeping is the sense of a responsibility for knowledge of one's origins.

This possibility of abandoning the reassuringly familiar to go towards the strange, the *Unheimlich*, can be seen as a sort of *unconditional hospitality of the mind*. According to Derrida (*De quoi demain… Dialogue*, 2001) it is expressed in momentary changes of direction when we are able to welcome the *Qui venient*, which I would define not as "that which may arise," but as the mental space – likewise unconditional – for taking a close look at everything surprising and unexpected that we are able to accept and welcome. If it actually happens, this does not depend on an external event but on being ready and willing to offer this unusual and impossible form of unconditional hospitality that only the psyche can give.

This scandalous patience – and I am thinking of the analyst's in traumatically repeated situations – is not to be understood as a continuously unconditional disposition, but as an exposure to being reached, which for Laplanche corresponds to the rejection of one's own knowledge and thus a listening more aimed at *taking in than understanding*; and *taking in* is a content of theory also taken up by Piera Aulagnier.

In conclusion I would like to mention *The Plague* by Camus. This great allegory composed in 1946–1947 does not talk about *an* illness but "*the* human illness" which arrives with the war, because of it and by means of it. (See also *The Triumph of Death* by Pieter Bruegel, mentioned earlier in Chapter III.)[12]

In *The Plague* some people do all they can to resist the disaster while others shut themselves in their houses; some continue to think only about their own interests, while others accept the plague as a punishment. And there are some who only manage to join the resistance later, once it has begun to make progress. Humankind is able to defeat its human illness by abandoning solitude in a collective operation that unites people and overcomes the epidemic through a paradox which inverts the plague's own logic of enforced isolation.

A brief appendix is needed to this concluding part of the chapter, a first draft of which was written a year before the book was finished. I included this part in other writings of mine as a comment – critical, of course – on the position many people were taking towards migrants, seeing them as an epidemic. In other words, this came before the explosion of the Covid-19 pandemic. Since then I have not changed a word and have no intention of doing so. I would just like to point out the need for some clarifications about isolation and collective participation. Imposed isolation – but also isolation chosen with immense conviction by many people – is necessary for containing the spread of an infection when suitable habits of hygiene are not rigorously respected in times of epidemic, and especially when there is a lack of sanitary, hospital, and regional structures proportionate to demand and an extensive need for vaccines. Nevertheless, those at home can work effectively with those outside. The many opportunities for electronic communication, resisted at first by many people, and still resisted by some, filled the gap left by the tragic alternative of a total lack of personal contact and enabled couple and group relations to be maintained. Of course this was possible along with, inevitably, the acceptance of a loss and the ability to mourn so as to avoid the omnipotent triumph of a personal viewpoint which some people continued to insist on, sometimes against all the evidence and at risk to their own and other people's health.

Thinking about psychoanalysis and sessions held remotely, the setting was certainly *varied*, otherwise it could not have been maintained: varied just as present historical reality is varied in an epochal manner if we *test reality* as Freud advised us to. In fact, if we denied this we would be seriously engaging our systems for denying reality. The setting was varied but not *transformed*, not denatured, attacked, or demolished: at least I hope not.

Bach's *Goldberg Variations* have often come into my mind, revealing a harmony of arithmetic and geometry in which the thirty variations inscribe two circumferences which revolve around distinct centres that are out of phase and yet maintain an indissoluble relationship with each other. Similarly, during remote sessions in that spatiotemporal phase-shift, patients tried to rediscover their setting, as did analysts; or so I can, and wish to, imagine. In this search for a new adaptation I thought something might be happening to both participants that was like what happens to dogs and cats when they go round and round on their cushion – familiar and yet unfamiliar because it has been displaced, washed, adjusted, but still with the same characteristics and use – before finding the right position and lying down, often with a big sigh of relief at the rediscovery. Once again, with Freud, is the object never found but always re-found? And isn't the setting also an object-investment?

I'll ignore the details of the *Goldberg Variations*, since structural analysis is tedious, just as I ignore the countless experiential details discovered by every analyst while they were confined, feeling the astonishment of a primitive child-man seeing the world for the first time and still capable of being surprised. Astonishment dazzles, surprises, and excites the first time, then it goes back into the frame that is established to define the event – into the setting, indeed – and it is right that it should, so that all the energy released by the astonishment can be channelled into thought. In the days of confinement and the switch over to remote sessions I thought about Freud's astonishment at the first use of free associations – the paradoxical norm of psychoanalysis: the rule of the absence of predetermined rules for thought – and I never forgot Green's observation, strongly maintaining that the setting is too little spoken about in the psychoanalytic literature, and I think he meant in theoretical-structural rather than dogmatic terms.

In this long/not long period of time I was often able to think again about the quotation from Camus, which I found in my first draft written during the pandemic. So I did not think of it as a prophetic idea – epidemics are part of human history; it hardly takes a prophet to think about them – but as a content that could be used as a metaphor for the most recent pandemic because one was the symbolic anticipation of the other. But there have been many "viral invasions" in the past few decades.

Widespread drought and humankind's great blindness about what is happening on our planet have made us unable to see that a human invasion – a matter of survival for a great many people, the migrants – could be the anticipation of other invasions with the same origin and cause: humanity's attack on nature, an attack that disrupts natural processes and accelerates abrupt changes which occur even when nature is less disturbed, and in turn disrupts the identitary processes of a suffering humanity.

Lamentation-Compianto

Their names are written on water
Desire is one axis
of the barge lashed by foam.
The blue a plastic bottle
floating on the wave.
The sky looks on with eyes of stone.
In the seagull's cry there is your name,
Dunya in the name the arms that weaken
your child. In the clamour of the sea
there is Mohammed, your name, and in the name
the bowshot of your running legs.
There's your name, Yasmin,
in the wind's voice, in the name your flashing eyes, the bitter
grace of your footstep.
The cliffs down there scream names,
in the names the shade of palm trees,
traders calling, caravans
in the night under worlds of stars.

The clouds' lofty indifference,
drunk with their flight to the east.

Antonio Prete, *Tutto è sempre ora* [Everything is always now], 2019

Notes

1 Some of the topics addressed here were previously discussed in Breccia M., "Identità eterogenea: Identità Personale ed Impersonale" published in an issue of the *Rivista di Psicoanalisi* with a focus on *Identità multipla, Identità eterogenea*, 4, pp. 745–755, 2018a.

2 In the work from which I have quoted, Stara refers to Starobinski's *The Living Eye* (1989) and his thoughts about Freud's *The Interpretation of Dreams* (1900). On the subject of knowledge, Freud is seen by Starobinski as the equivalent of Shakespeare's Hamlet. As Stara puts it, Starobinski takes up the interpretations of Hamlet by Jones, reversing the specifically psychoanalytic focus and emphasising that its subject is not the relationship between the drama of Hamlet and the biography of Shakespeare, but the relationship between their experience and the scientific life of Freud, creator of the Oedipus complex.

3 In this connection, see the article by Chiara Saraceno in *La Repubblica*: "Solidarietà e voyeurismo emotivo" (24 August 2019).

4 *Unheimlich* (uncanny, strange, unfamiliar): a term used by Freud in opposition to *heimlich* (familiar) in *The Uncanny*, 1919.

5 See also Breccia M., "Norma-follia-disseminazione" [Norm-madness-dissemination] in the section focusing on *Intersezioni* in the *Rivista di Psicoanalisi*, 3, pp. 753–760, 2020.

6 See the interesting book by Jean Paul Matot, *Le Soi disséminé. Une perspective écosystémique et métapsychologique* (2020) which, though it does not deal explicitly and specifically with identity, unites psychoanalysis with the ecosystem in a dialectic that renders them inseparable. It is also a reflection on the terms "dislocation-delocalisation" since in relationships they may become the central fact of the Self, an idea in tune with the thinking of Kaës in *Le Malêtre* (2012). I feel I must add that "dissemination" and "contamination" are also worthy of reflection because of their affinity with the recent pandemic and the persistent threat of further pandemics in the future. Covid-19 spreads from one subject to another – and before that from animals to humans, leaping across the species barrier – via small vital elements of the host's

body, reminding us how many parts of ourselves we disseminate in life and how both body and mind are contaminable, which obviously also brings fertilising and generative possibilities.

7 See Gaburri, A., *Pensare con Freud* [Thinking with Freud], 2013, but also Agamben, G., Nudities, 2009, which proposes that a purely biological notion of identity creates an "identity without a person."

8 See René Roussillon, *Agonie, clivage et symbolisation* (1999).

9 I am thinking of other examples which carry their own destructive charge and cannot be considered legitimate free expression because they threaten public health and safety: Covid denial and the anti-vax movement generally, and obviously the many forms of fundamentalism which suppress the education of women, such as Boko Haram and the Taliban.

10 See works by Primo Levi such as *The Drowned and the Saved*, Liliana Segre's *Fino a quando la mia stella brillerà* [Until my star shines], *Fatelessness* by Imre Kertesz, *Under a Cruel Star* by Heda Kovály, the five documentary films collected as *Shoah pour mémoire*, Vassily Grossman's *Life and Fate*, and many others to which I will refer in my chapter on genocide.

11 See again the article by Chiara Saraceno in *La Repubblica*, "Solidarietà e voyeurismo emotivo."

12 In his description of the episode, which portrays the consequences of the wars and pestilences of his time, Pieter Bruegel fuses two iconographic traditions: the Italian, in works such as the Palermo *Triumph of Death* (link indicated in the same note) which he may have seen during his visit to Italy in the mid-sixteenth century, and the *dance macabre* of Nordic origin (link also in the same note).

V

TRAUMATIC DISLOCATION

Genocide – *A brief introduction to the link between trauma and time, and a clarification about current history*

In a study about time in trauma I considered it essential to revisit history's great traumas, in particular the collective traumas that have characterised genocides.

We should not overlook the psychic dislocation inflicted on the Ego by a substantial trauma, nor its many repercussions for the single individual as well as for group and collective reality. Extremely large-scale traumas like those caused by persecutions and genocides, perpetrated according to perverse principles of annihilating the human, can in fact undermine the foundations of individual identities and those of the groups they belong to, an effect persisting over many generations.

However, what I find most disquieting and puzzling, and hence an ethical and scientific reason for study, is what goes before, not only in terms of the responsibility for causing genocides but, above all, because whatever is human can recur, as Primo Levi reminds us, and as we are tragically witnessing at this very moment. Indeed, in terms of racist persecutions, even in current history, there is a recurrent and disturbing oscillation between a reductionist or simplistic over-eagerness to compromise one's own belief and outright denialism. It is rare to come across hypotheses about how to stop such a dramatic phenomenon in time, before it reemerges with uncontrollable power, as it did in the past as the *Shoah*.

The study of History and histories is of course essential for the construction of future life and history, and as psychoanalysts we set

DOI: 10.4324/9781003747581-6

ourselves this challenge every day. And it is in everyday life that we hear echoes coming from the past. But perhaps this habit of repositioning ourselves makes us less unaccustomed to placing ourselves in the places and times where this abomination has been carried out so that we can set them alongside the places and times of other genocides and those of our own time. This may involve a habitual, and undoubtedly important, work in *après-coup*, but I don't think we should overlook the work to be done *avant-coup* as part of current history, the world's and our own. Such an effort is obviously not aimed at reestablishing a *quo ante* but at mobilising many psychic and methodological energies of psychoanalysis onto phenomena that are reappearing, circulating, and advancing in a far from subterranean manner in individuals and groups.

Current generations are still being struck by the humanitarian debacle that was Nazism and its contemporary, Stalinism – some directly as descendants of the persecuted, some indirectly – to such an extent that we wonder, as I found myself writing a few years ago, if we really can talk about a post-Auschwitz,[1] sharing this idea with Valeria Egidi, who left us in 2019 and whom I would like to recall here because of her cultural passion for these subjects.

As Julia Kristeva often reminds us, besides our feeling that we are training, theoretical, or political analysts, we definitely cannot speak only of analysts in the session but must also talk about analysts in life and – I would add – feel the responsibility of this.

I will try to examine the relationships between the individual, the heterogenous, and the multiple, and compare them with the idea of the collective. The path I follow will take in the psychic agencies, the drives, and the transferential and countertransferential elements involved in analytic listening to trauma, especially a great trauma like genocide, that is inflicted on humanity by another, dehumanised part of humanity.

However, I would also like to offer a reflection on the play of identitary mirrorings which, through various processes of identification which did not come to a good conclusion in the life story of the individual and their group, may suddenly explode and become a way to justify and legitimise expansive processes of aggression. This is all significant, in my view, because it constitutes an ever-ready *potential* for the perpetration of *collective traumas* – as I will continue to call them for now. My purpose is certainly not to identify an undifferentiated transversality of trauma but to seek the potential alterations in the identity of individuals, groups, and future generations which may derive from it.

According to the definition adopted by the UN, genocide means "acts committed with intent to destroy, in whole or in part, a national, ethnical, racial or religious group."

It was Raphael Lemkin who first introduced this term *genocide* in 1944 in *Axis Rule in Occupied Europe: Laws of Occupation – Analysis of Government – Proposal for Redress*, in which the author, of Jewish origin and a leading expert on the Armenian genocide, addresses the problems of Europe under Axis domination. His study reworks reflections previously made public in 1933 at the *Fifth International Conference for the Unification of Criminal Law*, which established that racist attacks had an international character, and the study of persecutions like those carried out by Nazism would help to construct a platform for the future legitimacy of all efforts to punish any crime against humanity. Little more than a half century later, all this seems forgotten, simply ignored; or perhaps, when we think about recent racially motivated crimes committed even in 2020 by the forces of law and order in the USA, it would be truer to say it is completely denied.[2] Still more recently, we have unfortunately witnessed the tragic situation between Russia and Ukraine, with many brutalities and atrocities that can be classified as war crimes, and the horrible Middle Eastern history that has driven the latest vile *pogrom* on 7 October 2023 by the terrorist organization Hamas and the unacceptable fury unleashed by Israel's government on the civilian population in Gaza.

The search for a name for unspeakable destructiveness inevitably prompts reflection. The term has a mixed etymology partly from the Greek *génos* (lineage) and partly from the Latin *caedo* (massacre), and only entered the terminology of international law and many national codes after the Second World War, being adopted at the Nuremberg trials in 1945. In 1946 the UN underlined the collective nature of "denial of the right to existence of entire human groups" and in 1948 it adopted the *Convention on the Prevention and Punishment of the Crime of Genocide*. In addition to the *Shoah*, the Convention has officially recognised the wars and genocides in the Former Yugoslavia, the genocide in Cambodia, and that of the Tutsis in Rwanda resulting from racial hatred between Tutsi and Hutu, a conflict that had not surfaced despite ethnic differences before colonisation by Belgium.

It is likely that events in various parts of the world, starting with what is happening in Gaza, will be classed as genocides.

There are many historical genocides, more or less acknowledged. It may be helpful to recall that during the colonial period and through the nineteenth century, whole indigenous populations disappeared for a variety of reasons, including forced labour: 90% of the Tahitians, 70% of the Kanak, and 60% of the Māori. The original Tasmanians have died out completely. The native populations of the Americas were reduced by around 90% during colonialisation. Among the often forgotten genocides are those of African peoples: the Congolese as a result of Belgian policy, the Sudanese as a result of British policy, and the Herrero of present-day Namibia as a result of German policy, and among Asian genocides that of the Hazara in Afghanistan. In the twentieth century we cannot forget the tragic extermination of the Armenians, the mass killings in China during Mao Zedong's agrarian reform and the Cultural Revolution, and the wiping out of the Kulaks in Ukraine during 1932–1933 at the instigation of Stalin, who starved the small landowners to death.

The *Shoah* remains incomparable, and we hope will remain so for the rest of human history, not only in the number of victims but in the strategy which sought out and persecuted even those Jewish people who were living outside the boundaries of the Third Reich.

Collective traumas are deposited in the territory of the unconscious and in clinical treatment of the *unsymbolised* pending transformation as it waits for an event located in a discontinuous and "de-affected" space, as Eva Weil reports.[3] A cultural event may be enough to do this, being collective and at the same time intimate, as is witnessed by several case studies of generations who came after the survivors. The cultural event can encourage the original traumatic event to emerge in the analytic process out of the psychic enclave in which it had remained enclosed, as if mummified, over a long period of latency, as Eva Weil (2016, 2021) again reports.

The subject who has directly suffered trauma or had it deposited in the unconscious transgenerationally seems able to emerge from *latency* through the presence and representability of a group and collective reality with which to identify, thanks to historical, literary or artistic testimonies and the possibility of using the analyst as a witness. Through a process of identification in which the symbolic is renewed, it then becomes possible for the subject to become their own witness. Thus it is a true work of *Kulturarbeit*: see Nathalie

Zaltzman (2007). This all entails the reconstitution of a psychic space capable of integrating historical lacunae and negative elements of the psyche such as denial and disavowal (which are inevitably also enacted and undergone on a societal level, and to an ever greater extent).

However, before a psychic space could be recomposed, the Ego had to deal with the breach of the para-excitatory system caused by the trauma and, using the analytic process, face the gradual emergence from traumatic repetition, which has an enormous range of expressions, almost always enacted – such as silence, for example: see Donnet.[4]

As I suggested in the second chapter of this book, repetition is not a sign of a predominant death instinct but of the Ego's struggle to amass all its resources to challenge it, and even though this effort does not guarantee life but only hypothecates it, it may nevertheless guarantee a prolonged survival. The deep harm done to the para-excitatory system, which, in Freudian theory, is located between internal and external spaces, compromises the separation and relationship between these spaces. But as a result it also compromises the possibility of representing them. An attack like genocide is the most shocking expression of this dislocation, decomposition, dismantling – and the most demonstrable large-scale instance of it – by which the Ego may come to be split off and inhabit a psychic space that contains a split object. The excitation provoked by trauma coming from both directions (external–internal), and no longer reined in or channelled, remains disorganised and disorganising to the Ego and its psychic functioning. As a result, phases of excitation may alternate with phases of absolute unexcitability, with a consequent diversion of the drive, as Bernard Chervet puts it, quoting Green on the *negative movement* of the drive.[5] Vitality is profoundly damaged or made rigid, more or less reversibly, both in excitation and in its opposite.

The attack on the single individual's para-excitatory shield also renders the "collective" sphere undifferentiated, homogenised because, once invaded by the energy of this charge, the individual extends it into the shared common space so that the charge's invasive element becomes pervasive. Kaës reflects on this as an important factor causing a rupture between the individual and the group. I will come back to this.

I do not share Primo Levi's view (*I sommersi e i salvati* [The drowned and the saved], 1986) that the real witnesses are the dead, nor am I entirely convinced of the case made by Nathalie Zaltzman (*L'esprit du mal*, 2007) that there is a collective Ego destroyed by the trauma of a genocide. In *De l'art à la mort* [From art to death] Michel de M'Uzan maintains that *death will be annulled if, "despite being dead, one can still interrogate the reality of one's own life*" (1977, p. 15, my italics). Embracing this paradoxical claim, I am more inclined to think that, instead of a destroyed collective Ego, there is a severely damaged Ego no longer capable of interlinking with the collective while differentiating itself as a single being, multiple and heterogenous. Only in certain rare cases is this Ego able to go on interrogating the reality – both historical and psychic – of its own life. De M'Uzan's claim is paradoxical, but fits well with the term *survivor* (from the Latin, *supervivere*, "to live beyond," "live longer") which is a living beyond the permanent certainty–uncertainty of death, an afterlife: but is it really still *a living*? The question interrogates the ambiguous and oscillating character of the survivor, still balancing between life and death because of the recurrent evocations of death which are persistent in survivors, and also because they strongly pull towards the past:

"With a shudder he pictured his mutilated corpse, lying motionless, at the mercy of the most abject of his survivors": so says Manzoni as his Don Rodrigo suffers a night of torment caused by an overwhelming sense of guilt about Lucia (*I promessi sposi* [The betrothed], chapter XXI, p. 309).

However, in the most severe and extensive traumatic experiences there is no possibility of giving meaning to a historical experience that the subject clings to like a survivor. It is in these extreme situations that there are sometimes two aspects, *personal and impersonal identity* (Chapter IV), looking for an identitary mirroring in the transference-object to guarantee their survival of the trauma, as well as a possibility of life in the future. This potential transformative possibility thus makes survival precious by its very ambiguity, because it has left a space open to the possibility of an *identitary becoming*: precious and also a threat if this becoming is halted, goes backwards, or is paralysed in an impasse with no future, in a counter-time set against living time.

I would like to offer some reflections about this fine crevice, this *shadow line* of survival which sometimes becomes an agonising crevasse.

In an exquisite work of history and autobiography entitled *Under a Cruel Star: a Life in Prague* (1941–1968), the Jewish Czech writer Heda Margolius Kovály (1986) makes clear the smoothness of the transition from Nazi tortures to those of a Czechoslovak regime totally subjugated to Stalin, a smooth transition that is naturally denied with no apparent sense of contradiction. This all happened not only because the population was the victim of an ideology of violent power but also for another reason: when a tyrannical system becomes dominant, the mere effort to survive is so strong that there is no way to evaluate errors further up the chain. As Kovály says, the only tranquillity such a climate could allow was to go to bed, happy not to have been taken away, arrested or dismissed from one's job – which at that time was equivalent to arrest. And of course this human poverty could make no room for solidarity or criticism, at least in most cases.

It is not hard to think that the climate of terror experienced by inmates of the Nazi extermination camps sometimes crushed all feelings except those of mere survival, at least for those long periods where the logic of survival had to predominate.

We have to remember that the re-actualisation of the past constantly threatens the present. Indeed, there are not so many differences for the inhabitants of Raqqa, including children, forced to witness daily decapitations and mass executions. But what more can be said about the atrocities being committed by the Israeli Army in Gaza? Among these atrocities we have to count not only the direct killing of civilians, but also deaths caused by the deprivation of food, running water, and electricity, or simply because hospitals have also been destroyed. Sad images of "human" madness.

Nor is it hard to conclude that current (and essential) logics of survival in relation to exigencies like poverty, unemployment, and migration induce adaptation, indifference, withdrawal into oneself, not only when external reality is atrocious but unfortunately also when it is deeply disappointing or frustrating: it is crushing in all these cases. This is how it was for many survivors of the Nazi extermination, as recalled by Primo Levi, Imre Kertesz,[6] Liliana Segre, Piero Terracina, and Hilda Hrabovecká, who survived three years in Auschwitz (1942–1945) and was the central character in Daniel Friedmann's documentary film *La dernière femme du premiere train* [The last woman on the first train] (2014), and many other witnesses like them.

According to Cornelius Castoriadis[7] we need to consider how, if society offers objects of identification with little significance for the subject, then if a subject adopts them, an economy and a dynamic are found which are proper to both, the social subject and society itself, and this is what fosters a continuity of pathological transmission.

We find some examples which contradict this in the various forms of *resistance* during the Second World War, of which an extraordinary example is given by László Nemes in his film *Son of Saul* (2015).[8]

Saul is a Jewish Hungarian deported to Auschwitz-Birkenau in 1944 and then recruited by the camp guards as a *Sonderkommando* forced to take part in the extermination of the Jews whom he accompanies on their last journey; then he is condemned to death as a witness of these crimes. He joins fellow inmates who will not submit and are organising a rebellion, and decides to recognise the corpse of a boy as his son. It becomes his inner mission to give "his" son a proper burial. In looking for a rabbi to say Kaddish, Saul will make a revolution of his own. He thus dies not by Nazi condemnation, but for having saved the body of "his son" with Kaddish and burial, and so he has saved himself and his identity, which enables him to await the death "he has chosen" in serenity and peace.

"*The readiness is all*" says Hamlet (Act V, scene ii) when he finally feels "ready" to accept the inevitability of death as decided by Divine Providence.

I recall that Kertesz meets persecution in the Communist regime of the East after that of the Nazis simply because he will not conform to one fate, as he emphasises in the title of his Nobel-prizewinning book, *Fatelessness* (1975). He does not want to write what other people want to hear him say about the Nazi persecutions: instead, he wants to describe how he survived by watching the beauty of the sunsets in Auschwitz, a beauty that sustained him in his *identitary resistance*.

And I like to think of other forms of *identitary resistance* in contemporary history as humanitarian rescue services on land and sea and as various kinds of reception centre.

What does psychoanalysis offer in this complex overflow of threats to and loss of identity? And what possible misunderstandings surround the term identity?

The first question we have to ask ourselves is in fact whether the current threat to/assertion of identity – a single supreme identity – may present us with a tragic repetition of recent history. Because if that is the case, we would have to believe that the individual and collective denials which wreck the memory of the past have invalidated the efforts and sacrifices made by so many people to bring an end to a past dominated by oppression.

Freud did not anticipate persecutory scenarios in the years when he was writing *The Future of an Illusion* (1927), *Civilisation and Its Discontents* (1930), and *Why War?* (1933), even though these were the years when Nazism advanced and finally triumphed in Germany. He did, however, aim to stress that the imperatives/restrictions imposed on the individual by civilisation (*Kultur* understood as a society's civilisation and culture) tend to bring about the explosion of something primitive (or perhaps it would be better to say anti-civilised) which may then triumphantly prevail and become racism, xenophobia, and war. His thinking makes us reflect on the various rebellions, those saying No, taking them as one example, however varied their motivations – among which we cannot ignore the economic. Freud's idea makes us examine how in these cases too there may be an intolerance of *Kultur*, seen as an unacceptable social hierarchy through which it is impossible to rise, or as a "caste"; but it exists nonetheless. Sometimes the explosion of the primitive is also provoked, more or less consciously, by an absurd competition between different interpretations of *Kultur*, disregarding the danger of the explosions this may encourage or trigger. On the other hand, the phenomena of splitting are no respecters of class, as the Schreber case clearly reminds us.

A minority may prevail over and oppress a recalcitrant and indifferent majority, as if the pleasure of destruction remained in a state of latency, waiting for a triggering event to make it reemerge. Even in his last writings Freud maintained a view that is neither persecutory nor pessimistic but free of illusions, aware of the subterranean destructive urges which persist in humanity.

What kind of analytical proposal, then?

The implementing of the Ego's defences in possessing the trauma, which I pointed out in the second chapter, may perhaps pass through a long transitional zone: on this see Eva Weil.[9]

And while we are still looking for new clinical and theoretical perspectives on the position of the analyst, how can we neglect *ethics*? Certainly ethics have a reorganising function, and the idea of an ethical seduction described by Viviane Chetrit-Vatine on several occasions[10] serves to show how this may nevertheless be libidinally invested and, I would add, also be attentive to inevitable influences from the Superego.

And perhaps it is here that we may encounter a variety of thoughts in a theoretical space that is both *transitional* and an *intermediary* between borderlands – internal/external, past/present, singular/multiple – but may also become an intermediary between primary and secondary, subject and group-community, personal and impersonal identity, "original" identity and the identity of one's chosen group.[11] This is also a *potential space*, which can initially be offered by the analyst. I feel I should add that, as well as this, we must consider the role of witness to the *identitary resistance* which the patient is engaged in for their psychic survival. It is not enough to offer a potential space if the analyst is unable to *remain* in that space, to remain an analyst in Pontalis's sense and thus to remain in the resistance that the patient is making.

Resisting and *remaining* are not alternative functions but mutually completing, and it is the offer of this very complementarity which releases the potential for cure.

Culture certainly has a fundamental role for the generations who come after the survivors of genocide, and metapsychology investigates how to locate culture in the analytic process. I think it is important to say that a substantial contribution may come from the ability of culture and psychoanalysis to complement each other, especially in some processes where the trauma of genocide has wiped out part of individuals' history, sometimes over several generations. In these cases, the psychoanalyst can utilise the patient's own culture, as is it variously presented during the session, as a valuable lateral transference supporting and standing in for missing parts that have been deleted from the patient's memory.[12] This is already happening in many cases, but analysts sometimes ignore the object of the lateral transference or simply have no theory about it: worse still, they may screen it with alternative theories.

Historical, literary, documentary or artistic elements can in fact multiply the transference to the outside world, but this way of functioning may be converted into a basis for the analytic transference. Analytic work which witnesses and testifies to the patient's *identitary resistance* to trauma may also cross this boundary towards representation and find *a way out of latency*,[13] making a transition hitherto avoided as impossible: mourning.

Mourning is indeed not loss of memory, but the exact opposite: the ability to remember because representation is already re-subjectivating historical memory.

I shall now return to the aspects of identity considered in these two chapters to address the more difficult transition: *the relationship between victim and aggressor.*

From what I said in the previous chapter about the heterogenous characteristics and multiplicity of identity, and in particular the dual feature of personal and impersonal identity in a state of conflict that is present to a greater or lesser degree in every subject, it is possible to speculate that the massive attack on individual subjectivity – all the more so if perpetrated against a very large number of people – may create a collapse of the single parts: individual and collective, personal and impersonal. This collapse may subvert the order of the parts in conflict, but it may also lead to the de-subjectivation of every feature of the identity, turning them into mass phenomena deprived of their individual histories (in both the oppressing group and the oppressed, as Castoriadis reminds us). For example, one may think one belongs to a certain nationality, or has a certain political idea or religion, be part of a certain ethnic group, while knowing nothing about who one is as an individual, or without knowing the history of the single subjectivity that makes one have that idea, or that religion, or that nationality or ethnic group, and no other. All of this may result from various possible traumatic scenarios, with genocide as the most potent example. The testimonies of Saul and Kertesz perfectly illustrate the rebellion and defensive *resistance* against this risk.

In these cases the collective is no longer a term that indicates the keeping together of different subjectivities, but may become "massified," annulling all differentiation and making individuals into Jews, victims, "exterminable," with pre-ordained fates, and no longer persons with different identitary features even if they have in common their sense of belonging to a religion, an ethnicity, a culture in which the single subject chooses to be recognised. And, besides the examples I have recorded, this may apply to any form of exclusion, marginalisation, ghettoisation.

The collapse of identity – effect and cause of an attack that annihilates the Ego – brings with it the use of more primitive Ego-defences to guarantee survival. This is testified by the accounts of survivors, and Eva Weil talks about these as she records the varied ways in which trauma is denied and/or disavowed in the analytic history of those struck by it. Elements of disavowal characterise the latency phases, a latency that is revealed as necessary to bring into consciousness the direct or indirect experience of trauma which passes through several generations (2000, 2021).

Observing the collective attitude that denies and disavows trauma, in *Life and Fate* (1980) Vassily Grossman investigates at length the systems which exclude reality. As he records, these systems kill actual human beings since they falsify reality, hide it, silence it, deform it by replacing it with an idea that is not the representation of reality but evidence of a delusion which can be constructed as a substitute reality.[14] We cannot forget what is unfortunately happening on the social networks. What was reported and feared by Grossman has become everyday life on platforms where fake news claims the right to circulate without hindrance "as a sign of freedom." A long chapter could be opened on this grievous *misunderstanding* of the concept of freedom. It is no coincidence that the European Psychoanalytical Federation (EFP) has chosen "*Freedom*" as its theme for 2025.[15] Here I limit myself to emphasising the term *misunderstanding* so as to leave ample space for thought to the reader. As is well-known, delusion is an idea whose degree of perceptibility is totally divorced from verification by the subject – always assuming there is still some internal perception – and it completely lacks the prohibition against action that is interwoven with the fantasmatic scene of desire. And so the idea, unperceived by single individuals, leaving them unable to recompose a representation of reality, is completely de-subjectivated, even though the delusional functioning obstinately maintains it. And perhaps the obstinacy derives from the feeling that one is slipping away as a subject and the obstinate idea is only an exhausting attempt to cling onto something in a slippage that nevertheless drags on inexorably. In this way the single human destiny loses its unrepeatability. As Grossman shows, "Among a million Russian *izbe*[16] you will never find even two that are exactly the same. Everything that lives is unique. It is unimaginable that two people, or two briar-roses, should be identical.... If you attempt to erase the peculiarities and individuality of life by violence, then life itself must suffocate" (1980, p. 19). Grossman's book also underlines how a point comes where violence stops being simply a means to cause harm and destruction and almost becomes a cult object and a source of constant exultation, sometimes unfortunately to the victims as well.

What is happening in the current wars occurring in such large parts of the world that is difficult not to think in terms of a world war is tragically continuing to prove Grossman correct. Indeed he reminds us that despair does not only generate rebellion but may also often generate the desire to be executed. In these words Grossman, who suffered long-term persecution like other writers such as Kertesz, demonstrates the broken equilibrium between good and bad, but also between the identities of the subject and the group, between the individual and the collective.

Therefore, "if you attempt to erase the peculiarities and individuality of life by violence, then life itself must suffocate," and the desire to be executed or execute oneself becomes massively true.

In the directory *Berlin in Zahlen*, published in 1949, the central office of statistics in Berlin records that in 1945 there were 7,057 suicides in Berlin. We must allow for the fact that after the outbreak of war the Nazis had suspended publication of suicide statistics, but even so the last figure published in the Reich's annual statistical summary was 22,273 suicides in 1939 (and this excludes those of military servicemen recorded in the rare testimony of the few Sonderkommandos who survived the concentration camps). The 1939 figure was followed a year later by a brief communiqué from the Wehrmacht offering reassurance that the percentage had fallen significantly (Huber, 2019).

For long periods of *latency* (Weil, 2000, 2021) the defences of negation, denial, and disavowal which decline to engage in reality-testing seem to be frequent defences common to the traumatised and their heirs, just as they are to a society that does not wish to feel responsible for the fact that previous generations have perpetrated the crime.

Angela Merkel only visited Auschwitz, for the first time in her life, in 2019.

A rejection of responsibility – the expression of a larger compromising of the psychic defences – involves those who were indifferent witnesses and want to deny their complicity, and may extend to the most delusional forms of negationism. Extensive evidence of this may be found in Pierre Vidal-Naquet's book *Assassins of Memory* (1987).

It is striking how far negation of the other's identity, which presents the other as an object of identification with little or no significance, is initially fundamental to the functioning of those who go on to perpetrate genocide, quite separately from the persecutory delusion which sustains the idea of genocide itself. We cannot ignore the fact that in the name of racial purity the Nazis put German children with Down's syndrome and other disabilities into the gas chambers, as Helga Schneider records in her memoirs.[17] It is at the behest of one unique identity that the multiple and the heterogenous are expelled from the psyche through a sort of abolition of internal perception[18] which, in my hypothesis, would go on to stretch beyond the single individual, as a result of which other single individuals re-entering the psyche from outside would be perceived as strange, threatening, persecutory, in an extended, and sometimes collective, plural paranoid logic.

The de-subjectivating "massification" may make the community adopt a similar economy and dynamic, and this cannot help but foster a pathological transmission.

If defences like denial and disavowal are common to both the victim and the aggressor, we have a duty to emphasise the complex qualitative and quantitative differences between the two. The concept of *identification with the aggressor* conceived by Ferenczi in 1933,[19] which was a thoroughly innovative metapsychological suggestion, must be extended by the advances in theory that link up with Ferenczi's idea and express the exceptional complexity of the condition in which those who suffer most extremely find themselves.

It is the trauma suffered in genocide and caused by a previously dehumanised desire for annihilation which determines an identitary dislocation and decomposition.[20] In its violence, this process of annihilation, structurally programmed in the case of Nazism though it was maintained by a *banality of evil* (Arendt, 1966), has interrupted the processes of symbolisation, threatening *identitary entirety* over generations, working silently, underground, and invisibly: with Yolanda Gampel (2006), we could even say *radioactively.*

Mourning endorses the possibility of "recollection" and in doing so, according to de M'Uzan, makes it possible to go beyond the trauma towards *a life preserved by means of continual self-questioning about it.* But mourning also endorses the fact of a legacy and a witness who must defend it, as Derrida (2001) notes. The legacy is what our predecessors have left us; the recipients find themselves faced with an unavoidable choice between two paths: one is to choose the part of the legacy which, responding to our subjectivity, feels as if it could belong to them, and thus to mourn for the rest. The other path is to testify responsibly about the chosen part, so as to keep it alive and pass it on.

I will return to the *ethics of responsibility* at greater length in Chapter VIII.

It is in fact easier than it may seem to pass from criticism of a crime to complicity in it.

In the museum founded on the site of the Warsaw Ghetto, one of the testimonies recorded there struck me in particular. The Polish writer Jan Błoński, perfectly summarising the concepts set out so far, says, "One may share responsibility for a crime without having taken part in it."[21] Here is an example of mourning as the overcoming of a trauma and a slow process of integration. The author, born in 1931, witnessed the phenomena of deportation to the Ghetto. His inability to help a Jewish boy who had asked him for help escaping the Ghetto tormented him for a long time with a feeling of guilt. But it later led him to work through this impasse by bearing witness to what had happened in the Ghetto, and across Poland, in all his writings.

While it makes as little sense to identify the nationality of a crime as it does to defend a nationality because we belong to it, it is nevertheless important and helpful to reflect on the ease of "complicity with the executioner."

> Without hair and without name
> With no more strength to remember,
> Her eyes empty and her womb cold
> Like a frog in winter.
>
> Primo Levi, Se questo è un uomo (1947)

Notes

1 See Breccia M., *Exilium: Oltre la psicosi* [Beyond psychosis], 2011.

2 The murder by suffocation of George Floyd at 8:46 p.m. on 25 May 2020 and the tragedies of Minneapolis.

3 Weil E., "Silence et latence" in *Revue Française de Psychanalyse*, 1, pp. 169–179, 2000. Weil E., "Traces psychiques, mémoires cryptées et catastrophes historiques," *Revue Française de Psychanalyse*, 2, pp. 488–500, 2016. "Lieu du traumatique, le génocide: Le nouage collectif-individuel" in the 80th Congrès des Psychanalystes de Langue

Française (CPLF), online, 13–16 May 2021, entitled *Espace psychique, lieux, inscriptions.*

4 Cf. Donnet J.L., Chervet E. et al., "La dramatisatio" in *Revue Française de Psychanalyse*, 5, pp. 1517–1550, 2015. Donnet J.L., *Dire ce qui vient; association libre et transfert*, 2016. See also Donnet J.L., *La situation analysante*, 2005.

5 Chervet B. et al., *Destins de l'autoérotisme*, dossier *Revue Française de Psychanalyse*, 3, pp. 609–717, 2018. The *diversion of the drive* to which Chervet refers is a drive movement that claims to reverse and bypass castration.

6 After surviving the Nazi regime, Kertesz was also persecuted by the Communists. His book *Fatelessness*, for which he won the Nobel Prize, was only published after the fall of the Berlin Wall.

7 Cf. Castoriadis C. *Socialisme ou barbarie*, 1969, *L'institution imaginaire de la société*, 1975, *La montée de l'insignifiance*, 1996, *All'epoca del conformismo generalizzato*, 1989, "La crise du processus identificatoire" in *La montée de l'insignifiance*, 1996.
"Le montée de l'insignifiance" [The rise of meaninglessness] is a concept also proposed by Kaës, in *Le malêtre* (2012), and reinterpreted by him as "the silence of those who do not respond to institutional automatisms" in the section entitled "De processus sans sujet et l'absence de répondant" [On process without subject and the absence of a respondent], p. 90.

8 For these and other forms of resistance to great traumas, see Natalie Zaltzman's theoretical concept of the *anarchic drive*: 2015, chapter 2.

9 See note 3.

10 Cf. Chetrit-Vatine V., "La personne de l'analyste ou… un espace matriciel pour M. E." in *Revue Française de Psychanalyse*, 68, pp. 1751–1757, 2004. In this paper the author takes Laplanche's concepts of *seduction* and matrixial space as her starting point for describing how the analytic encounter brings about a primal seduction which is re-actualised in the transference. It is in the primal seduction that the enigma of the other is discovered. See also Chetrit-Vatine V., *La séduction étique de la situation analytique: aux origines féminines/maternelles de la responsabilité pour l'autre*, 2012. See also Chetrit-Vatine V., "Toucher à la dimension d'infinité quand le sexuel est tout autant au rendez-vous" in *Revue Française de Psychanalyse*, 5, 2018. Lastly, see also the 80th Congrès des Psychanalystes de Langue Française (CPLF), held online by the Société Psychanalytique de Paris, 13–16 May 2021, entitled

Espace psychique, lieux, inscriptions in which she took part with Eva Weil to present the report "Espace psychique, lieu analytique, Makom."

11 A dualism which I have discussed with Silvia Amati Sas: see her most recent book, *Ambiguità, conformismo e adattamento alla violenza sociale*, 2020.

12 Psychoanalysis has been afraid of the lateral transference for a long time. In her presentation to the CPLF in Paris in 2017, Emanuelle Chervet challenged this by talking about the need for the analyst to use *bundles of transference.*

13 Weil E., " Silence et latence" in *Revue Française de Psychanalyse*, 1, pp. 169–179, 2000. "Lieu du traumatique, le génocide: La nouage collectif-individuel" in 80th CPLF, *Espace psychique, lieux, inscriptions.*

14 For example, "The pandemic does not exist."

15 EFP 2025 Dresden, Germany, 4–6 April 2025.

16 *Izbe* = huts.

17 Cf. Helga Schneider, *The Bonfire of Berlin* (1995), *Il piccolo Adolf non aveva le ciglia* [Little Adolf had no eyebrows] (1998), *L'usignolo dei Linke* (2004).

18 Indicated by Freud in the Schreber case (1910) as the basis of projection, a defence described there by Freud in the single individual.

19 What has happened in Gaza since the tragedy of 7 October 2023 strongly recalls Ferenczi's words.

20 During torture people reach an inhibition, also neurological, of physical and psychic pain. A person who cannot feel is like a person who does not exist. The subject does not exist and then the other can also no longer exist. This is how one patient described the dehumanization of violence. From my point of view this can be considered a confirmed and metapsychological integration with the concept of *identification with the aggressor.*

21 My translation.

VI

LIFE AUTOBIOGRAPHY – DEATH AUTOBIOGRAPHY

Autobiographical time

The case of Jan Błoński cited in the previous chapter is accompanying me as I ask the reader to consider some aspects of autobiographical writing and its unconscious variants, especially their implications for different timelines and their possible relations with instinctual movements.

Piera Aulagnier says that, in thought and in writing, one goes on looking for what has been left unanalysed in any analysis, which confirms the unconscious autobiographical aspect of all study and all writing; and writers such as Italo Svevo[1] have found a precious space for interiority in other kinds of writing.

I think of writing as the search for something left unsolved, a search that aligns with and relies on the libidinal impulse towards a sublimated object, an object deferred but comfortably at ease in the thought that sustains it while this unsolved remainder continues to accompany it. And so the use of writing to advance along the path of sublimation opens up not only a prospect of multiple scenarios but multiple possible versions of every single piece of writing.

I intend to dwell on these features in order to address both the idea of the multiple, which returns in these chapters, and its hidden temporalities, a multiple that multiplies the temporal possibilities.

Memoirs of My Nervous Illness (1903), introduced to Freud by Jung and used as the basis of Freud's *Schreber Case* (1910), is a well-known instance of autobiographical writing but it also shows how no piece of writing is ever destined to exist in a single version. I briefly refer

 DOI: 10.4324/9781003747581-7

here to examples from the bibliography of the Schreber text: *Soul Murder: Persecution in the Family* (1973) by Morton Schatzman; *The Schreber Case: Psychoanalytic Profile of a Paranoid Personality* (1974) by William Niederland; and Lacan's reading (*Le Séminaire, Livre III, Les Psychoses*, 1955–1956) which enumerates all Schreber's symptoms in a sequence between two poles. One pole is the *roar*, the pole of uttered sound and of the seduction attributed to God – the seduction of Schreber who feels he is God's wife – an uttered sound that precedes any elaboration in words and is thus the pole of the meaningless. The other pole consists of *the cries for help*, a pole centred on articulate speech which becomes an appeal to the Other. Schreber is undoubtedly the model for one of the most studied, discussed – and, I would add, rewritten – psychiatric cases of the twentieth century.

With regard to multiple rewritings, what I would especially like to keep in mind in these reflections is the fact that readers may draft their own versions as they read, versions which may already be potentially present in the text being read if the writer keeps the dialogue with the other person constantly in mind as a feature of all writing.

Leaping forwards in time, but also contextually and thematically, I now move on to cite André Gorz (*Letter to D.*, 2006)[2] specifically because he maintains that the inexorable presence of the Other makes the difference between being a writer and someone writing. On the other hand, writing is itself infused with such transformative elements precisely because of its "unreality," or rather, because of its characteristic of being – by means of the Other – the complement of the un-realising of the real,[3] and Imre Kertész confirms this in *Fatelessness* (1975) when he talks about the beauty of the sunsets at Auschwitz.

Art, and in particular figurative art, has always taken the possible plurality of a work into account, and that seems to suggest that this plurality represents a significant autobiographical element which can be extracted at every reworking, simultaneously transformed and transformative. (We can think of the plurality in Andy Warhol's works as an identity seen through a plural chessboard using the techniques of reversal painting and camouflage,[4] and at the same time as the expression of a profound autobiographical correspondence characterised by the great plurality of his artistic encounters.)

Indeed, the testimonial aspect of every artwork brings back into play the question of transformation, as opposed to the irreversibility of the work that remains, but this does not lead to an unresolvable aporia, since the aim is sometimes to leave several traces of a single process, several possibilities, which may be successive or contemporaneous, of an internal experience and its will – usually conflictual and ambivalent – to emerge: or perhaps it would be better to say "its emerging will." Art is thus the bearer of that heterogeneity-multiplicity of Ego-defences in a state of conflict with the Id and the outside world, which draw on a psychic heterogeneity (biology-psyche) together with the transformative possibility of its *becoming* (the Freudian *soll Ich werden*).

In the film *Le Mystère Picasso*, a biography-documentary from 1956 which won the jury prize at the Cannes Festival of that year, Henri-Georges Clouzot portrays one of the greatest twentieth-century painters in his studio: Picasso. Director and painter are both present as people and as characters in this presentation. Clouzot places the camera behind the canvas while lighting the canvas from the front, at the side the artist is painting. This enables the creation of the painting from the viewpoint of the subject while the *object of the painting* is being created. Above all, it enables us to see the successive transformations, since Picasso often chose to paint another picture over a previous one. The successive temporalities of the picture's transformative realisations, regrettably lost for those who see only the final version – as is the case with all transformed pictures – are preserved by the film, which becomes a living plurality. It does not avoid mourning but bears witness to what was there before and to the many creative and transformative possibilities that time grants to the painter and also in this case the viewer.

Picasso frequently declared that every picture has a great many pictures lying beneath it, the fruit of different nascent emotional experiences, but how can we fail to see the same goal in Caravaggio's use of light? The goal of making one part of the scene emerge to the viewer while the other also exists despite being effectively submerged in shadow and unrecognisable: it exists and is present at the scene of the other, illuminated part.[5]

In figurative art, certain self-portraits also reveal the simultaneous presence of transformative elements in a state of becoming, where we can detect not only the aim of self-representation but the fact that it is based on the artist's own reflected image and thereby presents features which reflect the artist's interiority.

Some other examples: Albrecht Dürer "presents" himself in a self-portrait which expresses his need to identify wholly with Jesus Christ;[6] Michelangelo portrays himself in the flayed skin of a martyr in the Sistine Chapel and again in the Rondanini Pietà of which he made two versions, working on one until a few days before his death, leaving it incomplete. As he left it, it shows him in the mortal remains of a Christ supported by a female figure, perhaps his own mother. In contrast, Francis Bacon[7] portrays himself as a deconstructed image which seems intended to correspond to the disorganising features of a psychic experience.

These extraordinary artistic outcomes have the power to help us think about the artist's reconstruction of their identity through the autobiographical trajectory of the artwork's realisation.

Nevertheless, the reconstruction of identity depends on the possibility of, or the subject's capacity for, self-historicisation – the *past of memory* – and the possibility of prefiguring an identificatory project that may be the anticipation of the future via the symbolic representation of the object-Ego in its state of becoming.

Here, using writing as my starting point, I would like to highlight not so much the flaws of such a project as the fact that it may be challenged by unconscious deviations under the sway of the death instinct. As an object of thought and as a thought-object, writing is subject to libidinal investment via the controversial function that is sublimation, which I will pause briefly to consider.

Freud addressed the concept of sublimation at various points in the reworking of his thought, from the 1897 letter to Fliess where he talks about it for the first time in connection with the phantasies of hysteria, to the 1910 essay on Leonardo where he explores his idea more deeply and indicates that sublimation is a third way after repression or the return of the repressed. However, he did not devote a paper to it specifically. Speaking about sublimation in *The Ego and the Id* (1923), he notes that the sexual drive makes great quantities of energy available for cultural and civilising work: thanks to sublimation, its goal can be displaced without reducing its intensity. Thus, for Freud sublimation is the ability to change the goal of libidinal investment by displacing it onto a goal *that has become related* to the object, no longer directing it towards an object in itself but towards an Ego-function relevant to it: knowledge. The point of origin posited by Freud is that the child is highly stimulated on the erotic level but does not discharge the drive onto the object, instead directing it, and thus transforming it, onto the epistemophilic passion.[8]

Further to "making the goal related" to the object, I like to recall the importance Green attached to the "objectivating function" of sublimation which helps to challenge the desubjectivating function (unbinding, *déliaison*) and the consequent predominance of the death instinct (*Key Ideas for a Contemporary Psychoanalysis*, 2004). On this subject Green proposed an interesting model of "character" which would essentially revolve around three elements into which he inserts sublimation: a degree of instinctuality which we could identify as both biological and part of the representational repressed (for example, the thumb being sucked by the foetus to activate several functions including the sucking that will be needed after birth. I would associate this with the aspects of the Ego *in fieri* noted in *The Ego and the Id*, 1923, although Freud could not be troubled as we are by the amazing ultrasound image of the foetus). Green goes on to note a reactive quantity of *counter-instinct*, a quantity of conscious Ego-defences which tell us little or nothing about the unconscious instinctual impulses and so may confuse us. Lastly, as a potential lifebelt, Green suggests there is a quantity of sublimation, highly variable from subject to subject and within each separate individual. This last element, though it inevitably depends on the first two, is nevertheless evidence of how much the Ego has learned to make good use of the object so that it can go on to use it as an object of thought.

Indeed, the fact that thought belongs to *being* ties it to *becoming*. Lacan very incisively reminds us that, contrary to some current translations of *wo Es war soll Ich werden*, curiously equivalent in several languages, Freud did not use the definite article *das* for either the Ego or the Id as he does in *Das Ich und das Es* (The Ego and the Id), and according to Lacan, Freud's aim is to emphasise the assertion of subjectivity *as it becomes* (Lacan, 1966, pp. 225–252).

So we could say, in addition to the classic translations, "where it was, I shall become."

Becoming can be considered a *potentiality that accompanies the Ego and precedes it*, and brings the subject up against the limits of knowledge within the "boundaries *of* the mind" and thus inevitably makes "boundaries *in* the mind" also emerge, with the real risk of ghettoising thought.

Dante makes Ulysses say, "*fatti non foste a viver come bruti ma per seguire virtute e canoscenza*" [You were not made to live as brutes but to pursue virtue and knowledge] (*Inferno*, XXVI, 119–120), and although Dante had very limited knowledge of Ulysses (from Ovid and Virgil), he could not help being fascinated by this figure who, in his desire for knowledge, had the courage to go beyond the Pillars of Hercules and face the unknown. Ulysses had to be placed among the damned for fraud – his deception of the Trojans – and because he was outside the Christian faith; and yet the words of Dante-Ulysses reveal esteem and admiration for a difference that can only be used to one's advantage by accepting the challenge of obscure and highly dangerous regions: a continuousness of thinking, entirely human, sought even in Hell.

For his part, Freud often plunges deeply into literature, drawing on the works of Goethe and Shakespeare, dipping freely into the Tales of Hoffmann and Biblical texts, and making no distinction between high culture and fairy tales or children's stories. He also makes constant reference to the scientific reports of his time and the findings of anthropology, a memorable example being *Totem and Taboo*, as I mentioned earlier in Chapter III. This tendency, which I find valuable for its transverse relationship with other disciplines, cannot, I believe, be attributed to an unscientific propensity on his part or to the controversies which psychoanalysis had provoked in this regard. Freud always wished that his theoretical and metapsychological hypotheses would receive scientific recognition one day. Even in my first reading of Freud I found that a great pleasure as a reader came from the author's extensive research since, in describing the object on a theoretical plane, the instrument he used was the very object he was describing: the libidinal investment of thought. Nor should we overlook the fact that Freud was awarded the highly regarded Goethe Prize for literature, as much for the scientific merits of his work as for its literary qualities.

Indeed, the literary text offers that plurality of voices that are so well-adapted to the possibilities of extended "sense" and "movement of meanings" in a state of becoming which are intrinsic to psychoanalysis.[9]

While sublimation maintains writing as a libidinal investment of the thought-object, it is also true that a sublimated, and thus in some way transitional, object may risk becoming a totally deferred object that in the end is unreachable. This may cause the investment to fall back onto the Ego, transforming the libidinal investment of the object into a narcissistic investment of death; and an example of this is Leonardo da Vinci, who abandoned painting because he thought he could never attain perfection in it.

Autobiographical writing can therefore also be subjected to the death impulse.

There are certainly a great many examples of autobiography in the literary sphere and some of them are mirrors of the suffering of those who wished to preserve a memory of their psychic experience, like the manuscript *Memoirs of My Nervous Illness* (*Denkwürdigkeiten eines Nervenkranken*) by Daniel Paul Schreber which I mentioned earlier.

In fact, some autobiographical texts seem distinctly more representative than others of the bipolarity that I am trying to describe in autobiography, texts where either the libidinal investment of life or its marked opposite is to the fore.

I am thinking, for example, of Strindberg's *The Inferno* (1897) set alongside *The Facts: A Novelist's Autobiography* (1988) by Philip Roth: a risky comparison perhaps, given the time span between the two writers, but it corresponds to paths of association travelled long ago and to which I have enjoyed returning as I reread the two books.

The Swedish poet and playwright August Strindberg, who lived during the second half of the nineteenth century and the early twentieth century, is less well-remembered than the celebrated Norwegian writer Henrik Ibsen because, while Ibsen became the apex of the Scandinavian literary tradition, Strindberg never achieved the same degree of literary success or popularity. In the end his marked and often irascible tendency to sociocultural polemic never brought him the fame he so desired.

Among his works, *The Inferno* is a singular and enigmatic book which does not yield to easy reading. The author drags his readers straight into the book's movement, even before we have had a chance to orient ourselves within it, which inevitably generates a resistance to carrying on. Indeed, I had the impression that I was walking through a hellish labyrinth where, however much I needed to find the way out, the tendency to give up and surrender was just as strong as a tortured curiosity about going further in.

I won't tell the story of *The Inferno* but, using some passages from the Afterword by Luciano Codignola, I will spend some time looking at points that I have found critical. The editor wonders from the outset what kind of narrative work this is: is it an autobiographical novel?

But if it is hard to track down the autobiographical aspect, apart from in the author's own declarations and avoiding banal detours, it is pretty much impossible to find the writing subject. The oscillation between reader and narrator is set in motion immediately, to dizzying effect, especially if viewed from within the extremely dispersed nature of the contents. After misadventures, tribulations, and torments, the narrator finally discovers that he is in hell. However, his hell is quite a particular one and rather attractive in a psychoanalytic reading, or at least it has been for me, since the narrator is always accompanied by a "mysterious friend" who helps and advises him from afar, even though the poor damned soul can never transform his condition. I firmly reject any tendency to clinical readings of a literary text, but Codignola's question about the autobiographical experience stays in the front of my mind; and the description of the friend offering advice from far away while nevertheless being powerless strongly reminded me of an *exiled Ego* (a condition which is present in a standard psychic equilibrium under exceptional circumstances, but frequent in psychosis. See Breccia, *Exilium. Oltre la psicosi*, 2011). The aim of the autobiographical aspect might seem to be the bearing of witness to a friendly, still living part (the Ego as a psychic agency) when everything threatens death, even though this friendly part is powerless inside the overwhelming experience.

In relation to the troubles experienced by this "missing subject," as Strindberg presents it, it is interesting to note that a Swedish edition of *The Inferno* runs to three volumes, while there is a French edition in four volumes. An examination of the texts shows that he sometimes speaks in the first person and sometimes the third, and only in the final book of the French edition does he return to the first person "I". This has led me to think again about his experience of writing, divided between several representational possibilities, as an attempt to put various versions of the Ego into operation through writing without arriving at an integrated result, and therefore with a "missing subject."

One can write the same way one lives, and Strindberg, who lived on the run, wrote on the run. His writing thus seems to be the instrument of his flight and at the same time the attempt to contain himself.

So writing is not only an attempt to contain the trauma which may have been the impulse behind the writing, nor is it simply the testimony of one's existence and the need for it to be said and written; writing seems to be a necessity in itself. Codignola says very appositely, "But what matters is not that *The Inferno* narrates an experience, reproduces a pulsation: it is that pulsation" (*The Inferno*, 2012 [1897b], p. 404). As Strindberg says in his attempt to cajole his persecutor, "Interned in this little Town of Muses, without hope of getting out of it, I engage in the terrible fight against my worst enemy – myself" (The Inferno, 1913 [1897a], xiv) and then, attempting to attack the enemy and trying to destroy his phantasmatic power: "What is one to do then? Humble oneself? If you humble yourself before men, you will arouse their pride, for all will think themselves, no matter how guilty they may be, better than you" (The Inferno, 1913 [1897a], xiv). A mask of falsehood, however damaged or corrupt, may be the only possible condition for the Ego's survival in the hope-uncertainty of a future where some redemption may be possible: "The sun shines, everyday life proceeds on its usual course, the cheerful bustle of business raises the spirits. Then one feels rebellious, and challenges heaven with doubts" (The Inferno, 1913 [1897a], xiv).

But there is never a glimpse of this future in Strindberg's book: the attempt at a vital experience that might overcome the persecution seems inexorably to fail and the autobiography seems to be deposited in his story like a plaque commemorating a redemption which life had perhaps not given him. The book is dominated by a backward gaze: there is no progress in using experience as a way to look ahead, and no growth of creativity. What predominates instead is opposition to the judgements imposed on him, accompanied by the ambivalent need – one that cannot be suppressed – to lay down his own laws about truth, which sometimes leads him to lose contact with reality.

To me, Philip Roth's experience seems the exact antithesis of this. *The Facts* has an illuminating subtitle, *A Novelist's Autobiography*, and it introduces us to the paradoxical aspects of this definition, as the author is keen to make clear from the outset in the *Prologue* and in the *Letter to Zuckerman*, one of the figures who have often represented him autobiographically in his novels, especially in *The Counterlife* (1986).

In *The Counterlife* Roth claims that while he was writing he could not see exactly what he was doing. By contrast, in *The Facts* he seems to see the work from a distance and realises that the manuscript does indeed represent his true counter-life, both an antidote and a response to all those inventions of his writing, culminating in *the invention of himself.* So he thinks that if in a certain sense *The Counterlife* can be read as a fictional structure, the *facts*, which are his autobiography, represent its bare bones. With great determination and a considerable degree of introspection Roth examines the reasons for his move into autobiographical writing: emergence from a state of psychic illness that he calls "nervous exhaustion," not so much an account of how the pathology had gained the upper hand and how he had nevertheless survived it, as how writing had been not merely a testimony but the means of combatting psychic pain. "Insofar as the rest of me, which had collapsed as well, intuited that stripping the writing down to unvarnished specificity was a part of getting back what I'd lost, a means of recovery and a way to strength, there wasn't even a choice. I needed clarification, as much of it as I could get – demythologizing to induce depathologizing" (*The Facts*, p. 7).

Always highly attentive to his inner experience, he adds:

> This isn't to say that I didn't have to resist the impulse to dramatize... to abandon the facts when those facts were not so compelling.... But on the whole it was easier than I thought it would be to escape from what I'd felt constrained to do nearly every day of the pre-crack-up existence.... The nonfictional approach has brought me closer to how experience actually *felt* than has turning the flame up under my life and smelting stories out of all I've known. I'm not arguing that there's a kind of existence that exists in fiction that doesn't exist in life or vice versa... but simply saying that a book... that leaves off with the imaginative fury, can unlock meanings that fictionalizing has obscured, distended, or even inverted and can drive home some sharp emotional nails.
>
> (*The Facts*, p. 7)

And as he further clarifies: "Obviously the facts are never just coming at you but are *incorporated by an imagination* that is formed[10] by your previous *experience*" (*The Facts*, pp. 7–8, my italics).

However, the central feature, formidable in its incisiveness, lies in the final questions he asks himself: "why should anybody other than me be reading it?... especially as this feels like the first thing that I have ever written *unconsciously*" (*The Facts*, p. 9, italics in original). And again: "Is the book any good?... I'm in no real position to tell" (*The Facts*, p. 9, italics in original).

I found Roth's expression "counter-life" poignant because his use of *counter* seems to be in tune with what I am proposing about *counter-time* in this book.

Roth claims that in his autobiography he is telling his real counter-life: that is, his life as a novelist in which he had to invent himself.

Does that perhaps indicate that this self-inventing was a counter-tendency or a compensatory wish for not feeling himself?

Was self-inventing perhaps a way to survive in order to see himself and to be in the future, only at a later time? Perhaps it was a moment when he could discover the desire to tell his story through autobiographical writing which, nevertheless, if it is to be true it is always transformed because "the facts are never just coming at you" (*The Facts*, p. 7).[11]

What I pick up in his words about the presence of other people in his writing is the essence of my own thinking: that a *life autobiography* always includes the Other, cannot exist alone or for itself, and that this is not only participation by the Other, but its becoming – in other words, the possibility of infinite new versions of thought and at the same time the future and the vital continuity that goes with it. This is the presence which makes possible the *un-realising of the real*, exploiting that embodied imagination which, challenging the imaginative fury, leads back to a previous experience and transforms into a legacy of testimony left to the other and to the future.

While Roth's text is an autobiographical model of his becoming, Strindberg's instead seems constantly subjected to the desire to actualise the autobiographical project by making its *sublimatory inactuality* fail.

This specific outcome seems to link with the interesting article by Sophie De Mijolla-Mellor, "Specificità dell'autobiografia del paranoico" in *L'Autobiografia Psicotica* (Balsamo, 2015). Keeping a sublimated object alive seems in fact to be very difficult in psychosis where the object is fused with its maternal complement, as Sophie De Mijolla maintains; or, as I have often found myself thinking, where an object is confused with the totalising object proposed by Green,[12] as I noted in Chapter II, and hence in agonistic and antagonistic relation to it. All of this hinders or obstructs a recognition of feelings of identity.

According to Sophie De Mijolla what appears to be impeded in schizophrenia acquires sense in paranoia, where it may even be possible to find a real need for autobiography founded both on the necessity of self-justification in the face of imagined or delusional accusation and on the megalomaniac desire to take oneself as a model. The autobiography would thus fulfil an identity-forming function, even if pathological, for the additional reason that every autobiographical undertaking requires the subject to situate themselves paradoxically on a timeline, which is well-suited to the paranoid state.

By fixing their story in a text which, from the moment it is written seems to evade movement and the uncertainty of becoming, the autobiographer could use the text to find that fixity, that immobility of self-image that he or she seeks.

I think De Mijolla very effectively captures certain risks of autobiographical writing, but I would add to her findings that there are nonetheless several different ways out, even in psychosis. In fact there is a multiplicity of forms – in a state of becoming, indeed – even within the most challenging pathologies, the complexities of which can be detected and explored in clinical work. In analytic practice there is always an open dialogue with doubt, as there is in any proposition awaiting verification, a doubt that, as we know, destabilises every positive assertion that is instead aimed at an operation to do away with a part of reality. In paranoia it seems impossible to accept *precariousness and waiting as necessary conditions for movement.* Mourning is impossible to deal with.

It is certainly true that death introduces an irreversible change, the ending of the living subject: nothing more can be added to that life and those lives. But is it really true, outside its unquestionable materiality? The fact of death certainly interrupts a physical existence, but what remains are the thoughts offered to the outside world and other people for adoption or as a legacy; and, as Derrida says, if a legacy is to be passed on it must be libidinally invested and thus in some way reacquired, as I noted in Chapter V. In the end, don't we do this every time we theorise? Doesn't the "thought without a thinker" find in a thinker a new, innovative way to express itself?[13] Didn't it already exist elsewhere in another way of thinking?

Nevertheless, while it is true that a thought can only be autobiographical, autobiography or a piece of writing that preserves autobiographical features is something else, and the work of Sophie De Mijolla helps us to rework some reflections deriving from this difference.

As I said when I introduced this chapter, autobiographical writing presents two possibilities of development which I would regard as two opposed vertices. The first pole starts from a retrospective view, from an afterwards that addresses a before. It only looks over its shoulder and wishes to tell the story of the life that has been lived, fixing it in reassuring certainties. In this case the position would be that of the dead person who wants to tell their life story, a life already passed.

This position is liable to quite a few pitfalls: for example, the illusion that writing from the dead can vividly pass on the life being described and recounted along a more or less definite timeline; or the illusion that the reader takes this rigid version as sole truth and does not instead detect the hypostatic, unliving tracks onto which they are dragged by the act of reading. I believe we can recognise this tendency in the autobiographical accounts written by difficult patients in psychoanalytic treatment: in other words, the aim of the assertiveness and definiteness is to render the self-image irrefutable and unmodifiable, hypostatic. An immediate objection might occur to the reader: these are stories that happen to have been written down rather than stories *by writers*, and the sphere of observation and reading is primarily clinical, and therefore related to a symptomatology. I add furthermore that the reading of these scripts cannot happen in the analytic setting: the analyst only listens to their story, but psychoanalysts who work in the public services have testified to the frequency of these writing exercises.

So differences exist and must be kept in view: the paranoiac's enlightenment, based on which the entire meaning of an existence is "re-signified," is a highly distinctive characteristic of these needs to write.

There are autobiographies which have nevertheless found a place in history, such as those of Hitler,[14] Schreber or Wilkomirsky,[15] which are strongly characterised by this hypostatic aspect and at the same time by its denial, because they strongly express the wish to maintain the idea of the thought and the narrating subject as alive, whereas everything in the books is not.

Together with the blocking of becoming-time, there is a prevalent wish to bend time back onto its past, which is associated with a parallel desire to arrest history and its truths.[16]

What also stands out in these autobiographical models is a wish to render the reading subject passive, blocked from being able to participate actively instead of passively, or simply forced into rebellion, but never involved in a constructive relationship between writer and reader. In these testimonies we do not feel even an attempt to work the mourning through: indeed it is negated and in its place appears the megalomaniac effort to keep a false image, rather than a recollection, alive by fabricating a memory that is often projected and resists yielding to reality-testing. Reality-testing would inevitably cause separation and loss, and – because of what is missing – would on the contrary allow the gradual freeing of the recollection which must lose the concreteness of its "reality" if it is to find its place in memory.[17]

As I have already emphasised, this extreme position is probably to do with a profound alteration in the recognition and development of the identity, and hence in the ways it is claimed and communicated. It is as if a sort of collapse occurs between *idem* and *ipse* – the same and the identical[18] – resulting in an inability to develop a difference between the identity articulated according to multiple facets of the narrating subject and the subject's narrative identity.

By contrast, this indispensable difference is made vividly apparent by Philip Roth in *The Facts* with great refinement and literary sensitivity, as well as a capacity for introspection.

Sometimes, in still more extreme cases, this collapse coincides with an attempt to repudiate the past, to scotomize completely certain aspects of one's life and the relationship between selected facts and responsibilities that result from these. In this regard, Hannah Arendt's account in *Eichmann in Jerusalem: A Report on the Banality of Evil* (1963) is exemplary. In this historical and documentary record of the Eichmann trial Arendt sheds light on the accused Otto Adolf Eichmann's absolute blindness in analysing his own responsibilities, together with his need to recognise himself in an *antihistorical historicisation*, as Pierre Vidal-Naquet would say. The story he tells is stereotyped and hypostasised, an account in which there are no questions that the subject could ask himself about his conscience as a soldier and a citizen – or even as the human subject of his own ethical thinking: there is nothing but the "execution" of orders. As well as denial, there emerges an almost delusional re-signifying of his commitment to carrying out his orders: getting rid of Jews to give them a better life, for example. And this aspect of the denial associated with delusional re-signification of what has happened is observed by both Arendt and Vidal-Naquet who, despite not being psychoanalysts, clearly grasp how denial comes to be one of the defences employed by those whose starting point is splitting and so are to a large degree psychotic, which does not by any means absolve them of the various kinds of negationism in their historical responsibility. How much denial and *antihistorical historicism* of every kind is present, and becoming ever more widespread, in the historical events of this moment is an insistent thought which not only worries us but makes us question ourselves in our clinical practice and in life.

In connection to this, I want to add that Hannah Arendt is an exemplary writer – and I would like to emphasise *writer*, and not just the fact that she was a journalist of exceptional quality – since through her writing and Eichmann's biography she is able to convey the history of a people, the Germans, the history of the peoples subjugated by them, and the story of a people persecuted to the point of genocide: the Jewish people. And so she is also able to write her own history with an extremely wide and expansive vision. In addition, she is able to show with invaluable vividness how the traumatic element can confuse the human mind and may lead to mistakes being committed in the name of justice and to deeds which, even if they are carried out according to the dictates of justice, will have negative long-term repercussions, essentially because they submit to political viewpoints, even before the ideological. How true and current her view is at this historical moment of war between Israeli government forces and the Palestinian people. Rereading her 1964 text we also glimpse a vivid capacity for foresight about what has since led to the tragedy of Al Qaeda and then DAESH. Clearly, the question of Islamist terrorism is multifaceted and complex, but this farsightedness is surprising, and equally surprising that it was ignored at first and even condemned by some.

So should we use the past as a shuttle to imagine a possible future? Perhaps.

Whatever the case, I believe that this is a matter that concerns analysts since, by making their wide range of functions available to everybody, they could participate with others in the effort to understand things that have happened before and so could happen again, as well as what is happening now. Because the difference – and the conflict – between the need for an irrefutable view of oneself and the desire, however much it is challenged, to surrender to a transformative possibility both belong to mankind. And also because, as Julia Kristeva reminds us, every analyst is also in history and not just in the session.

By putting together this heterogeneity and temporal multiplicity we can have a better idea of the short step between the desire to put oneself out of time, to rest in the illusion of being able to tell one's story as if in a freeze-frame, and the ambivalent, simultaneously present desire to recover a space in the mind which, in thought and in writing, may be able to pass through the boundaries of time without altering them.

With regard to the two potential types of autobiography – *death autobiography, life autobiography* – I also feel the need to point out that the two positions are never so precise and mutually impermeable.

While some of these undertakings are indeed a rejection of the irreversibility of passing time with the unconscious intention of stopping it, this is not infrequently associated with the desire to precede it, to go beyond, and not necessarily into death: to precede in order to go further, towards the future, a future freed both from the rhetoric of progress and from loss of contact with one's origins. It is from this viewpoint that Piera Aulagnier, starting with her experience with psychotics, emphasised in *Les destins du plaisir* (1979): the need for the Ego to be immediately recognised by the mother as something other than a pure repetition of herself; without such recognition the Ego would be left with the impossibility of thinking about a future time since it would only be recognised as the repetition of another person's past, anchoring it to a time before it existed.[19]

Every analyst can testify to clinical experience of this access to the future by the identity in a state of transformation, and likewise to the fact that the imagination, on loan to the tertiary functions of the analyst's mind, sometimes stands in for parts which history ungenerously failed to restore to certain subjects. The aim of this loan is to give back a "sense" which may enable the subject to feel the physical and biological sensoriality of his or her thinking and existing.

Reconstructions of this type, which sometimes also latch onto a transitory narrative identity, may therefore find, or lose, their most complete form in autobiography. The dividing line is fine and the window for passing through it is brief.

The Ego needs some self-knowledge, a sort of intuitive trace of itself, even when not involved in any actual autobiographical undertaking.[20] Our self-perception is most often achieved by default – and for unconscious reasons, to avoid conflict – by eliminating what does not satisfy us. In other words, this is a selective, and therefore defective, perception which operates more often than we might think. Maybe we can go along with what Philip Roth says about the novel, seeing it as a way to bypass a more directly autobiographical form of composition.

In the end, repudiating historical autobiography in favour of novelistic storytelling enables one's life story to be legitimised in another way, to edit out unwelcome things, overlay it with a different patina, and to tell the story in the guise of other characters. This is an aspect which Roth does not condemn but which, because of the significance it has assumed in *his* story, he finally chooses to move beyond, to go further.

Narrative identity, which also finds one of its expressive possibilities in analytic work, although it cannot definitely coincide with it – as is the case, in the end, with all aspects of evolving identitary feeling – may find its most detailed and coherent expression in autobiographical writing,[21] or it may just leave incomplete testimonies.

As the idea of writing presents itself in the analyst's mind, this incipient sublimatory process sets itself in motion with all the implications on which I have tried to shed light and with all the threats and challenges that are inevitable if the text is to come to life.

> The eyes are
> long strips of sand
> verges unmoving in the wind
> changing eternal, dunes.
> Still on the eyelash
> I chew its danger
> furrow of infected light.
>
> Vittorio Lingiardi, *La confusione è precisa in amore*, 2012

Notes

1 Cf. Italo Svevo – aka Aron Hector Schmitz, *La coscienza di Zeno* (1923).

2 André Gorz, born Gerhard Hirsch, was an existentialist philosopher, a close friend of Sartre, an anti-individualist and ecologist. He was born

in Austria to a Catholic mother and a Jewish father who changed his son's surname to Horst to protect him from growing anti-Semitism.

3 I think I must clarify something that may seem obvious but when I have mentioned this author on other occasions – at conferences and in writing – I have been challenged by some psychoanalysts who insist that psychoanalysis is concerned with "reality." Gorz is a philosopher, not a psychoanalyst, but I think it is part of the psychoanalyst's role to translate the language of the unconscious, and hence the language of the other. I cite André Gorz because I have found his thought to be very close to psychoanalysis, and certainly not close to what many people would consider an out-of-date psychoanalysis centred on the intrapsychic: I wonder what kind of psychoanalysis has ever been concerned only with the intrapsychic. I have cited Gorz for precisely the opposite reason: for the complementarity between the phantastically unreal and external reality, which is always translated into an inner reality and is the basis on which every psyche moves successfully forwards. I do not think there is any need to remind the reader how engaged Freud and most post-Freudian literature are with phantasies and their controversial interchange with reality. The British literature and those of other languages have done the same: I am thinking of Melanie Klein but also of Winnicott's *Playing and Reality* (1971) and his concept of sublimation and creativity. And, making another change of theoretical direction, we can remember the two-way movement indicated by Bion between conscious and unconscious, the residues of thought which produce the unconscious (*Learning from Experience*, 1962 and *Transformations*, 1965), and what Ogden picked up from this theoretical position in his suggestion that we learn to produce the unconscious, so to speak, by dreaming " 'The music of what happens' in poetry and in psychoanalysis" (1999); *This Art of Psychoanalysis: Dreaming Undreamt Dreams and Interrupted Cries* (2005). Obviously every translation is unfaithful, always interpreted, but isn't this a primary role for a psychoanalyst?

4 Mecacci A., *Introduzione a Andy Warhol*, 2008.
Reversal painting is an artform achieved by applying the paint to glass, which is then turned around so that the image is viewed through the glass, an ancient technique reintroduced in the eighteenth century on the mounts made by Jean Baptiste Glomy, hence the term *verre églomisé*. *Camouflage* in painting is a technique which renders bodies transparent, scarcely visible, by creating a blurred edge around the silhouette in such a way as to reflect the setting completely.

5 Cf. Caravaggio, *The Calling of St Matthew*, 1559, Cappella Contarella, Chiesa di San Luigi dei Francesi, Rome. https://commons.wikimedia.org/wiki/File:The_Calling_of_Saint_Matthew-Caravaggo_(1599-1600).jpg

6 Albrecht Dürer, *Self-Portrait in Fur-Collared Robe*, 1500, Alte Pinakothek, Munich. https://upload.wikimedia.org/wikipedia/commons/6/68/D%C3%BCrer_-_Selbstbildnis_im_Pelzrock_-_Alte_Pinakothek.jpg

7 Francis Bacon, *Self-Portrait*, Madrid, 1992. www.google.it/url?sa=i&url=https%3A%2F%2Fadierre.wordpress.com%2F2009%2F12%2F24%2Ffrancis-bacon-autoritratto%2F&psig=AOvVaw2EM3URUN_0BoXTVkAUvb0y&ust=1628952360922000&source=images&cd=vfe&ved=0CAsQjRxqFwoTCOCHj9CervICFQAAAAAdAAAAABAD

8 See also the "*un-active*" (i.e., neither current nor involving action) aspects of sublimation suggested by Rossella Valdrè in *Sulla sublimazione. Un percorso del destino del desiderio nella teoria e nella cura* [On sublimation: a journey through the destiny of desire in theory and treatment], 2015.

9 And which Lacan, in a definition that is entirely specific to his theoretical thinking, would call a *chain of signifiers* (1971, 1974).

10 I would add: *Formed* by your previous experience and *deformed* in being represented. Cf. Breccia M., *Rosă, Rosae, Rosae. Déclinaison-Construction-Déformation* in *Revue Française de Psychanalyse*, 2018b.

11 This inevitably links back to André Gorz and to note 3, both in this chapter.

12 Green, *Le temps éclaté* [Time in psychoanalysis: Some contradictory aspects], 2000.

13 This is what Claudio Neri wrote to introduce his seminar at the CIPA (Centro Italiano di Psicologia Analitica) in Rome, December 2006 entitled *Pensieri senza un pensatore* [Thoughts without a thinker]: "Bion opened the seminar held in Rome on 15 July 1977 with these words: 'I will begin by thinking that when there are many individuals present, there are also many thoughts without thinkers and that these thoughts without thinkers were, therefore, in the air somewhere'" (Bion W.R., *Bion in Rome*, 1977–1983).

14 In 1930 Hitler's *Mein Kampf* (1925) was being sold for 12 marks, printed in the same format as the Bible and given as a wedding present to couples in the Reich.

15 Binjamin Wilkomirsky's *Fragments: Memories of a Wartime Childhood 1939–1948* is a fake. It was written by a Swiss, Bruno Dössekker.

Despite the fraud, it won the National Jewish Award for Autobiography because it was only in 1998 that Daniel Ganzfried published the author's true identity in the journal *Weltwoche*. Dössekker was not Jewish and had not lived through the *Shoah*, as he falsely claimed. Following this, the German publisher Suhrkamp withdrew the book.

16 See Vidal-Naquet in Chapter V.

17 In this chapter I have intentionally omitted autobiographical texts such as those of Primo Levi, David Grossman, Liliana Segre, Heda Margolius Kovály, and many others which I have already discussed in Chapter V on genocide. The legacy of witness left by these writings, a witness that calls upon us all to make it endure, is located, as it is easy to intuit, in autobiography of life.

18 As I discussed in Chapter IV, together with other theoretical references concerning personal and impersonal identity, and as is also hypothesised by Sophie de Mijolla, 2015. It is quite clear that in this context, where there is a need to reintegrate personal and impersonal aspects of the identity, *idem* and *ipse* are used in a different sense from de M'Uzan's when he writes about the possible different characteristics of repetition in "*Le même et l'identique*" (1979, 2017) considered earlier in Chapter II.

19 I will return to these elements in Chapter VII.

20 On this topic, in Breccia M., *Le parole ritrovate* [Words regained] (2006) I hypothesised a transitory phase of this self-perception, the *existential Ego*, which is later totally absorbed in the fact of existence.

21 A further example, among others, is the character of William Stoner in John Williams's novel of 2012.

VII

CROSSING TIME

Historical temporality in "psychotic potentiality"

The Franco-Italian psychoanalyst Piera Aulagnier, founder of the *Quatrième Groupe*, constructed the concept of *psychotic potentiality* through a long process of clinical research while also developing a broad theoretical outlook that never abandons Freudian thinking but integrates it, making it complementary to other theoretical lines of thought, including her own, which is of course also greatly enriched by engagement with the Lacanian school in which she held a training role before breaking with them entirely.[1]

Her thinking is as rich as it is complex, and immensely helpful for anyone approaching clinical work with psychosis, but it can also be considered a foundational element in psychoanalytic training overall since it provides theoretical and practical methodological tools which support the analyst in clinical situations that are not yet manifest but still subterranean: psychotic potentiality, in fact. These are situations where the trainee analyst in particular would feel much less well-equipped without this support. Naturally Aulagnier is not the only researcher who has addressed the problem of a psychosis that is not entirely evident, but she is the only one who has used the concept of *potentiality* to help us see the transgenerational roots of psychosis and its various possibilities as actually a potentiality for development.

So Piera Aulagnier's concept of *psychotic potentiality* is more innovative than it may appear and different from other concepts that may be better known, such as Melanie Klein's idea about the mingling of two positions (the paranoid-schizoid and the depressive[2]), Bion[3]

DOI: 10.4324/9781003747581-8

on the "psychotic and non-psychotic parts of the personality," and Tustin's[4] "psychotic nuclei"; all of which are in their different ways circumscribed by a comprehensively non-psychotic functioning, or one that has the possibility of being non-psychotic. What differentiates Aulagnier's innovation is her idea of a functioning that refers back to early moments of psychic life which would remain silent but have specific structural characteristics distinct from other pathological constellations and, because of these, the appearance of critical events in the subject's external life may or may not allow the expression of a psychotic experience.

The concept of *potentiality* is important because it sets up a tension in the state of becoming – the oscillation between silent and manifest pathology and between pathology and "normality" – and thus makes extremely direct demands upon the analyst. These demands extend to questions involving long-term outcomes, not just for the patient in treatment but also for future generations. The weight of responsibility which all of this entails may mobilise an instant defensive disposition in the analyst, and it will be important to return to this.

But the feature of Aulagnier's thinking that chimes most closely with the subject being addressed here is the topic of temporality.

I have called it *crossing-time* with the intention of expressing a temporality cutting across the other temporalities: historical, biological, psychic, existential.

Aulagnier's thesis concerns something that has indeed arisen traumatically but has remained unknown, secret, and goes on to be silently passed down through several generations, *crossing a time without time* and without history.

Analytic treatment may enable the psychotic explosion to be avoided, both by defusing the explosive threats and by reconstructing the pieces of a history, and sometimes constructing them for the first time; pieces of history which time, without historical time, seems to have swallowed up. And the two things necessarily go together since it is precisely this deletion of a piece of biographical history – a deletion which endures over many generations – that is silently transmitted.

So I would like to revisit Piera Aulagnier's thought to rediscover the theoretical and clinical foundations of psychotic potentiality, a definition which derives from her research. The path I follow will not involve a close commentary on her thought, which I will cite briefly here and there: instead, I will follow the traces that I have found significant in my clinical work so that I can use them to delineate the concept of *psychotic potentiality.*

Aulagnier's observation compels us to reflect on the fact that psychotic thinking sets non-evidence against what is evident, since psychosis highlights the *less* of every existential story which addresses this experience. Hence the effort it takes to think about the *more*, especially the invasive excesses which the subject imposes on the other and which *The Violence of Interpretation* (1975) regards as inevitable, rather than pathological, in every child's development in the original relationship with the mother. Aulagnier's thought is thus prompted to explore a *psyche located "before"* the advent of the Ego, so that she can examine its origin.

This is why Aulagnier imagines three states of psychic development: *Originary*, *Primary*, and *Secondary* – something both more than and different from Freud, for whom Primary and Secondary are characteristics of the psychic processes which have a *locus*, an economy, and a dynamic: but this is all quite different from Aulagnier, who regards them as structural states of development. Freud makes reference to the *original* in the drive model, attributing repression to it: the original repression as a sort of great magnet (which is how I have always imagined and described it) that fosters and attracts towards itself all the processes of secondary repression, setting up an indispensable psychic dynamic that is unfathomable but always active.

And so for Aulagnier the *Originary* implies a *quo ante* of representation which, in this phase, knows nothing about a psychic outside and is therefore built on a supposed autogeneration. The *pictogram* is the element that characterises it, an element of representational activity that is definitively precluded from the knowable, as she calls it, and thus prior to all phantasy activity. It is a "putting into representation" of the psyche itself, although Aulagnier later opted instead for the term "presentation." And so this state is precluded from speech because its material is exclusively the *bodily thing* and it is as if it were at the same time setting up a structural background for the representation to come.[5] The background, though excluded from consciousness, would continue to function in all the other states and would be synchronous with them, just as the relationship *between* each of them always is. As I see it, this also takes the heterogeneity of all psychic productions into account, and is entirely in accord with Freud, who nevertheless follows other avenues in support of the background activity: unconscious representation and its investment by the drives, for example.

The *mouth–breast* contact would thus produce a representation that excludes an outside-itself, which would cause the breast to be considered autogenerated by the mouth. This is a proto-inscription perceived psychically as an autogenerated source of pleasure built on a bodily sensoriality in which an erogenous zone and its complement (mouth and breast, for example: see Tustin for this definition) are identified and go on to correspond to a function, a taking-into the self and an expelling-from the self.

But if there is unpleasure in this primal function derived from contact between mouth and breast, hate is activated. In these cases the *pictogram* may invade the scene and turn it into the drama of a body devouring itself. Thus, during its development the Ego will only be able to defend itself from this encroachment with delusion or with *speech-acts*.[6] For Aulagnier, when something of this kind happens during a session the analyst finds herself hard pressed in the countertransference since contact with one's own *originary* is equivalent to a difficulty in representing and even picturing it. (Remember the image of the mist in Tarkovsky's film, *Stalker*, in Chapter II). It's like being faced with a milky fog, a total whiteout, with faces all the same as each other:[7] life's potentiality for difference is diminished. But this raises some puzzlements and questions.

For Aulagnier, the *Originary* corresponds to something undifferentiated or a tendency towards the undifferentiated. As happens when the death instinct predominates?

This would seem to contradict totipotentiality, which is indeed little differentiated but nevertheless propels an emerging life. Perhaps, reading the author's words carefully, the emphasis should be placed on the tendency to return to totipotentiality, which indicates a possibility of lapsing into the undifferentiated.[8] However, an interpretation posited in these terms, even if motivated by the attempt to render it as metapsychology, would alter Aulagnier's idea. She is not thinking in terms of regression but of invasion; an invasion of the Ego's structure by a stage in which an *inadequate metabolization* (differentiation?) has not enabled the construction of firm boundaries to prevent it. This pervasiveness deconstructs, disorganises, and makes continuous that which should remain segregated, bounded, and mute.[9]

By contrast, in Aulagnier's theoretical vision the *Primary* corresponds to the representation of the *phantasy* which contains within it the omnipotence of *the desire for the Other*,[10] including the Other's body, and thus the existence of an external space. Passing from the previous state to this one necessarily implies the representational possibility of a separate body, and so the world of representation is already in operation.[11] This perception of the Other's omnipotence can only be rendered tolerable if the growing child is always allowed to preserve a *secret space*. It is this hidden separateness, protective and indeed secret, which enables the manifestation of thinking and the ability to keep drawing on it. It would be as well to stress that in this case it is not a matter of a gift being bestowed by the Other, but an attainment by the subject who goes beyond the Other while still being unable to do without the Other. Indeed, all of this can only happen if the Other is willing and able to allow it.[12]

For Freud unconscious phantasies are based on repressed elements – including among these the primal phantasies, which are objects of transgenerational transmission. They therefore remain as bringers of satisfaction for unconscious desire as well as being limits to its realisation. The phantasies are thus differentiated from delusion and hallucination because the subject is not alienated but is their author, included in the scene – as Winnicott also observes[13] – a scene that limits the desire to the plane of reality, shoring the subject up in this way against the risks of alienation.[14] The phantasies are still located between the subject and the object, between an internal world tending towards illusory auto-gratification and an external world onto which the subject wishes to impose the reality principle through the mediation of the perceptual system; therefore they are also located between phantasy and memory.[15]

For Aulagnier the space of sharing with the outside world is subject to the desire for the Other, as a result of which the outside world, as represented in phantasy, is more circumscribed, and also because the pleasure principle finds an obstacle in the Other and is overwhelmed by the omnipotence exercised by and attributed to the desire for the Other. In spite of the threat it implies, this "outside" continues to preserve the possibility for the *infans* to project its desire, and it also becomes an invaluable environment for illusory construction to compensate for a lack.

When she was a child, a patient of mine always used to say to herself, "Then everything will pass away and change and I'll find what's not here now," and for a long time that "then" remained her *phantasised temporal place* where everything could magically and in an illusory way be put right with a minimal contribution from her. The subject is always included in the phantasy scene, and connecting the past to the future is often a way to make the present liveable.

The *Secondary* corresponds to the *representation of the utterance*; in other words, an ideational representation which must draw on speech and therefore be comprehensible in the dialogue with the Other and capable of being built on that dialogue. By being linked to words, the representations of something participate in a perceptual quantum: mnemic traces/residues, probably auditory in origin.

Being bathed in the mother's language, says Aulagnier, surrounds the word with a persistent sensoriality since, as she herself will come to say, the sense of a word precedes and anticipates its meaning because it is a sense of acceptance and rejection. And this concept will be taken up and extended by Green in his definition of the halo of speech.

The possibility of abstraction is often diminished in psychosis because of a laborious and sometimes vain attempt to stay attached to reality, often merely imitating it to avoid it. But in a good situation for psychic development abstraction may be a way to keep control of reality, to manage, interpret, and utilise it with benefit for the subject who knows how to use it.

The question of parental love, which at first seems self-evident in the child's eyes, later becomes an enigma because of its erotic current, which overwhelms the child who does not yet have any means of decoding it. The enigma prompts and agitates the epistemophilic drive to know, which may thus be extended to investment of other areas of knowledge.[16]

The *states follow one another* in a process of *irreversibility* (which also seems to be a residue of the Lacanian school in Aulagnier's thought).

The succession just described is imagined as happening along a small gap which allows the process of *metabolization*[17] to come into effect. However, in the end the various stages coexist, even though the transitions between them remain inaccessible to consciousness.

How then, according to Aulagnier, does the Ego acquire a structure in this developmental process?

For Freud the succession of psychophysical experiences of the external world – when the encounter with it is good enough, we might add with Winnicott – enables them to coagulate onto the Ego, fostering its capacity for developing certain functions, beginning with that of representation. Then, as is well-known, the Ego finds itself performing a constant work of mediation between boundaries: those of systems, of agencies, and thus of definitions of every kind. The processes of identification and the good control of them inevitably lead the Ego to a constant work of renunciation and mourning for all the urges it might have had for expansion, for extending itself without limits and overflowing its boundaries: all of this happening while it is being integrated and applying itself to this task in relation both to the other agencies and to the outside world, but especially to the parts that constitute the complex heterogeneity of the Ego itself – psychic and corporeal, conscious and unconscious.[18]

Like Freud, Aulagnier starts from the study of pathology to imagine a non-pathological functioning, and she starts in particular from psychosis. The Ego is tasked with representing reality in a form coherent with the Ego's own structure, and this is in fact one of the aims of metabolization: to transform all information and render it coherent with the structure of the system that must receive it; in this case the Ego, which constitutes a system of functions that are coordinated in the present and on various temporal axes simultaneously. In Aulagnier's theoretical treatment of them, the first forms of representation are the *pictogram* and the *phantasy*, while the last is *utterance*. The Ego that she talks about is an Ego included in a temporality that is defined by means of temporality itself: the *crossing-time* I am proposing here.

In this concept of temporal crossing, its original interpretation is not so very far from the well-known and previously mentioned assertion by Freud in *The Ego and the Id* (1922): *Wo Es war soll Ich werden*.

There is thus always a "before" and a "where," a "where something was," and in Aulagnier's thought all this seems to be condensed into the *originary act*, which represents the mother–child encounter. It is also an encounter characterised by *heterogeneity* since it happens between a *mother who is the word-bearer* and an *infans* who has no speech, but it is an encounter that can become good if one party offers what the Other desires, and the Other has a desire if the first offer has been a good one; that is, if it has satisfied the need and thus fostered the establishment of the bases for desire. It nevertheless remains an *asymmetrical* encounter since it is impregnated with the mother's repressed sexuality and this leaves a residue in the *infans*, an *enigmatic representation*. (See *The Unfinished Copernican Revolution: Selected Works 1967–1992*[19] by Jean Laplanche for a helpful comparison of the differences and similarities with Piera Aulagnier's thought, but also to appreciate the rising spiral of concepts in the work of Laplanche.)

The *originary act* is a foundational encounter because it introduces word-representation through the anticipation of the maternal word and hence, with it, the function of language. The mother, who is therefore bringer and founder of the *infans'* language, is also the representative of *primary violence*, a constitutive and inevitable violence, but not therefore necessarily the harbinger of a bad mother–child encounter. This is why Aulagnier calls the mother the *spoken shadow*.

Her use of the term violence indicates the asymmetry and disparity of that encounter, which introduces a gap that remains permanent but, in good circumstances, is also a constant source of interaction.

Only when faced with excesses that do not allow this interaction and increase the discrepancy, widening the gulf of difference to the point of oppression, can we talk about *secondary violence*, which for Aulagnier is what leads to psychosis.

The Ego is immersed in this *utterance*, a world that speaks *to* it, but unfortunately and inevitably also *for* it, and occupies a space libidinally invested by the mother who makes herself the *word-bearer*. The term used by Aulagnier is *bouche-oreille* to indicate the closeness, almost the oppressive sensory intrusion, together with the corporeal-sensory circumscription that will open the way to the psychic. The Ego's capacity for projecting itself into the future – the *soll Ich werden* that begins with the use of these instruments – will be the guarantee of existence.

While for Freud memory and recollection do not go in the same functional direction – the former conservative, the latter transformative – *historicisation* becomes constructive where there is a memory of the events; but it also happens through the process of self-historicisation in the analytic work of reconstructing certain missing elements.

What, therefore, are the fundamental moments and transitions which allow the slippage from primary to secondary violence, and what features of those moments can specifically incline development towards psychosis?

But above all, what is it that sets up the psychotic potentiality? What blocks it, arrests it, and holds it back while at the same time letting it operate as the residue of a threat below the surface, and sometimes deeply submerged?

While the *originary act* defines the birth of a mother–child encounter, the *identifying act* defines the birth of the Ego which may find a conflictuality in this phase that may eat into the processes of identification and create the bases for a psychopathological development.

I should add that, in Aulagnier's view, the process of identification is not conflictual in itself, since it is once again anticipated by the *identifying function of the speech-bearer*, the mother, who was previously the *spoken shadow*. It is she who determines the *identifiers* that are offered to/imposed on the child, and with which the child must compare himself. As a result of this, the structuring of the varied potentialities for the *infans*' psychic development will be based on the available range of possibilities for identification.[20] Among these the most advanced is *symbolic identification*, which, for Aulagnier, is the real project of openness to the *identifiers in other people* – the processes of identification in others – and paves the way to the "*narcissistic contract*."

The name *narcissistic contract* – taken up and extended by Kaës – indicates the quality and weight that the social and the transgenerational have for the neonate, and it is summed up as the task imposed on everyone to ensure continuity in *that* generation, continuity *between* previous generations and that present one, and hopefully continuity *with* those to come.

It is a contract between the subject – still a child – its family, and the social whole in which both are immersed. Every subject thus has a place and a role in a society whose values, ideals, and cultural bases they agree to share. Therefore each individual within this reality proceeds along a pathway of subjective structuring, but for that to be achieved it is fundamental that this *intergenerational chain* can narcissistically invest the individual with the further role of carrying the chain into the future. And so the *narcissistic contract* ensures an origin and a continuity, but also ensures that, thanks to this investment by the group, the child has *the right to occupy a place independent of the parental verdict* (cf. Aulagnier, 1975, p. 214), a fundamental factor for projecting oneself into a historical and future dimension that will be able to relativise the maternal and paternal knowledge and desires, though without ignoring them.

When the *narcissistic contract* fails, the developmental process shuts down and changes into a sort of *pact* – tacit and in some situations forbidden – which effects a separation between the family nucleus and the rest of the social whole, both when the family excludes the social by closing in on itself – into its own myths and certainties, into its experiences of threat or its paranoid fears of exclusion – and when the social is deficient or excluding, persecutory, marginalising, or ghettoising, and in this way casts doubt on the social and cultural values of that family nucleus.[21]

This all unbinds the individual from their social group, and from previous, present, and future generations, suppresses their cultural values and encourages a superficial, regressive spontaneity, aggressive in its effrontery and arrogance – and sometimes idealised as sincere and authentic – which prompts and maintains the infantile feeling of omnipotence.[22] On the other hand, the child is immersed in this cultural order from birth because it is into this that the *word-bearer*'s language is rooted.

It is easy to understand the difficulty and conflictuality of maintaining the *narcissistic contract*, even when the most extreme conditions are not involved. However, its safety is the precondition for the survival of the subject, who may otherwise feel killed, as in psychosis, or threatened with death as happens in *psychotic potentiality*, a state of which we are given a fine and comically tragic example in *Through the Looking-Glass*, when Alice says "somebody killed something"[23] and the monstrous "something", the Jabberwock, could be a feared part of the father or of the child himself.

And this killing can happen very early on.

Setting out her reflections according to three parameters – need, desire, question – Aulagnier makes us *hear* – to use a term dear to her – rather than *understand*, how these three elements are inseparable in the child because they lay down the bases for a single purpose. *Need* concerns the state in which the absence of the object leads to a life-threatening condition. Indeed, the absence of food would lead to death because food is a necessity for life. For Aulagnier, *desire* is the psychic metabolization of the object of need; indeed the breast is not only the dispenser of milk and calories, but also of pleasure.[24] *Desire* is the advanced psychic state of need since it feels the same satisfaction in being gratified as it feels deprivation when the gratification is missing. We can add that desire understood as *mentalised need*[25] is the testimony of a need previously satisfied in all respects, and it is therefore also the search for a pleasure to be rediscovered because it was enjoyed before. The *question* at the beginning of life, the one we are pursuing through this author's thought, is an element integrated with the first two, need and desire, but it comes from outside because the mother is the interpreter of the question and she could partially distort both the need and the desire and thus also the question itself. For Aulagnier any question attributed to the *infans* is one that, besides the explicit object of the need, indicates *love as supposed by the mother* to be the object of that psychic need, and so the question offers the child a knowledge anticipated by the mother, the woman who offers love. An inevitable ambivalence in the mother is therefore implicit in the way the *infans* interprets love because of the vexations he may inflict on her, an ambivalence which, being perceived by the *infans*, may be translated in him as, "My mother asks me to need her love. Therefore I need her love because she asks me to."

Only if the child can assert his right to occupy his place in the future will he then be able to make the register of *Being* separable from that of *Having*. What the Ego becomes, what it believes it has become or desires to become, or what it would like to refuse to become, will also therefore always be the expression of a loss since this is the sole condition of a becoming capable of ensuring that the change which the Ego is trying to put into effect does not become synonymous with a deletion (that early killing of subjectivity I referred to above in connection with Alice).

The assertion of the *right to transformation* obviously implies that the Ego has achieved a condition of non-dependency and may therefore be capable of creating a series of safe references for itself so as to make a *judgement about existence* (to be considered, in my view, as an expression of *reality-testing*); otherwise it must be obliged to formulate this judgement using only the guarantee given by the Other – i.e., the mother – so that it becomes the mother's judgement transposed and stuck onto it. If this were to happen it would not be a transformation but a mere repetition and a subjugation: that is, another desubjectivating experience. Hence the importance of the father in this transformative process, and of other adults with auxiliary functions since, once again, the child cannot access all this on its own.[26] But the transformative process cannot proceed in the first place unless a reciprocal (and, I would add, recursive) process is set up to promote the *identificatory investments*: the child's in the adults, and thus the adults' in him.

In *L'Apprenti historien et le maître sorcier: Du discours identifiant au discours délirant* [The apprentice historian and the master sorcerer: from the discourse of identification to the discourse of delusion] (1984), Aulagnier described her highly metaphorical hypothesis of the mechanisms involved in the transformative process for the independence of every individual, the risks and their possible consequences, risks which later in historical evolution will come to threaten or compromise the *narcissistic contract*.

In this work she introduces the concept of *potentiality*, referring to the metaphorical image of the *jigsaw puzzle*.

While the mother must inevitably provide the first pieces of the puzzle – since, as Aulagnier will say, no autobiographical picture, no self-portrait, starts from a completely blank canvas – the mother also provides the first instructions about how to put the pieces together and complete the puzzle. Then the child's task will be to go on and choose the other pieces for building up a sort of family portrait, which must respect a certain order if it is to assume the correct configuration. So the choice of the pieces will not be entirely free since it must reflect an established order according to a law transmitted by the familial system over several generations. That locates the protagonists in precisely this order. Moreover, the pieces must have surfaces well-adapted to each of their slots, with no irregularities, and no pieces can be missing. Furthermore, the frame of the puzzle must be solid and stable enough for the pieces not to lose their position as the new ones are added. Naturally the new pieces will only fit in, not just if they comply with these preconditions, but also if they find a harmony, though not a homogeneity, with the basic configuration, so that the new pictures do not clash with the rest of the representation that has been put together.

However, it may happen over time that a seemingly perfect puzzle cannot keep its pieces together: if, for example, a piece slips from the picture, possibly revealing other holes until the entire picture is threatened.

This is the condition of *psychotic potentiality* and it is here that the *narcissistic contract* has probably been weakened right from the outset.

In Aulagnier's view, this *potentiality* weighs on the subject as a constant threat, and it is this sense of threat that explains the obstinacy with which the subject tries to make sure nothing changes, specifically so that the outcome of the whole construction is not irremediably compromised. To stop this happening it is necessary to prevent any change in the affective investments that bind the characters of the puzzle together and ensure that the characters guarantee the illusory certainty that this organisation of relationships always remains identical.[27]

The threat becomes a risk of catastrophe at precisely the moment when an external element begins to compromise this setup. It may involve an encounter with another person in whom the now adult subject affectively invests before realising that the place where the other person is located and locates the subject requires a repositioning that is incompatible with the original schema. Or it may involve a tragic loss, such as a death. Or there may be a sudden and unexpected change in a relationship. At other times the subject may have to deal with a change in their body image: pregnancy, for example, or losing or gaining weight, or an illness. All these situations make the ongoing change visible by means of the body.

The risk of passing into full-blown psychosis is no small matter if such threats interpose themselves into the rigid schema required at the start of life.

In this book, Piera Aulagnier makes an important claim to which I will return: she reminds us that generalisations in psychoanalysis are always arbitrary – and I stress the term *arbitrary* since, in my view, this risk applies equally to any generalised classification of the psychic. The denials of the claim when it is applied to psychoanalysis leave us even more convinced that it is true.

Despite that proviso, Aulagnier decides to advance along this precarious ridge, facing the risk of generalisation and pointing out two features that are often found in these subjects, using the experience of her numerous clinical encounters:

- The presence of *an event lived like a catastrophe* which prompted the request for help. And in this experience of catastrophe there is often a discrepancy between the scale of the event itself and the patient's lived experience of it.
- The *quality of the affective responses*, characterised primarily by the experience of persecution, unlike every neurotic or depressive reaction where the prevailing emotion is rage, despair, fear of rejection, or guilt. The patient then risks responding to this

> persecutory experience with a highly projective reaction which may lead to flight, increased aggression, or delusion, as if a fault line had suddenly opened up between the world of relations with the Other and the world of the processes of identification that have clearly already been threatened to an extreme degree.

It is at this point in the analytic process that the importance of *historical construction* becomes clear in all its intensity. *Historical construction* becomes the source of belonging-to-being and is situated between a mutually questioning past and a present, a state of conflict to which the Ego is nevertheless compelled to refer as the sole condition for its continuance.

I would add that this is how the subject, having "landed" in its historical and social reality, is projected towards a becoming that asserts its autonomy but at the same time is also the witness and heir of its history.

The *historicisation of a past* that is inevitably gone, its presentness lost, is fundamental if that past is to exist in recollection and thus form part of psychic life, while always being autobiographically recomposed and always revisitable.

But to guarantee the good cohabitation that is needed between permanence and change, it is also necessary for the subject to psychically recover their own *points of reference*, those that Aulagnier calls *funds of memory*, on which historical memory is founded and by which the reliability of the mnemic references is guaranteed. These fundamental traces have a safeguarding role, ensuring that change does not threaten the subject's singularity and unique character and – I would like to add – ensuring an acceptable level of coherence and unity between the parts that compose identitary multiplicity. It is by means of the *funds of memory* that the subject lays down a solid bridge to time past, in particular to childhood, which is stamped by the first representations and processes of identification that later become the basis for transformations and for the experience of mourning, repression, and recollection. But, above all, it is by means of these *funds of memory* that the affective resonance – both of the past and as it is being lived in the present – is transmitted and goes on to help in establishing that heritage of phantasy which safeguards the possibility of representation and thought. *Funds of memory* thus guarantee the reconstruction of a past which is where the cause and origin of our existence dwell.

Like any psychic process, the process of historicisation cannot do without the experience of relationship with the Other which, as I noted earlier, in Aulagnier's view violently anticipates the process in the figure of the *Other as speech-bearer*, the Other who fosters the actuation of a dependency from which, as I have mentioned, the subject can nevertheless make themselves autonomous.

For Aulagnier it is fundamentally important to refer to the paternal function at this point, not only because of what Freud has to say about it – that the father intervenes in the maternal dyad and effects the passage through the Oedipus complex by separating the child from its primary objects and introducing it to the search for an objectuality represented in the social – but also because the paternal function is what it is by being immersed in the social. The *narcissistic contract* firmly establishes the importance of the historico-social in the structuring of the subject by maintaining this contract and implanting the transgenerational passage in it.

Autonomy in choosing the pieces of the puzzle is not the representation of an unbridled individualism which, as I stressed in Chapter IV, often actually coincides with a dependent conformism, but is the result of a continual reworking and maintenance of this contract which operates by asserting the desire of a subject in a state of becoming. Consequently, its failure becomes evidence that the subject has lost all autonomy and all desire to become; and survival is only possible through a rigid and crystallised repetition of schemata which, if compromised, may later lead to psychosis.

I again briefly note, following Aulagnier, that maintaining the *points of reference* in the narcissistic contract depends on repression having been adequate, at least to some degree, since a deficiency sets back the investment of desire in the future while an excess may confuse the rediscovery of the reference points, as if the recollection of experience were flowing too quickly through the hands and slipping away like sand.

The conflict between object- and narcissistic libido is thus always open and subjected to the threat of the death drive.

Catherine Chabert takes up some aspects of this body of theory in an essay entitled "Piera Aulagnier: 'se construire un passé'", in *Topique* (1, pp. 113–127, 1992), a collection in memory of Aulagnier containing reflections from well-known writers including André Green, Sophie de Mijolla-Mellor, Nathalie Zaltzman, Guy Rosolato, Jean-Paul Valabrega, and others.

Chabert especially emphasises how the area of relationships is conditioned by and dependent on the quantity of identificatory positions the Ego can continue to occupy, on condition that these positions are also maintained in the transformed Ego. As Chabert interprets Aulagnier, this is in close relation to the link that will have been created between the various new relational phases that the child-subject moves towards and the phantasmatic representations the child makes, particularly with regard to their affective resonances. This operation – which, in my view, evokes the metaphor of the *pointe de capiton* proposed by Jacques Lacan[28] – allows representations to share their material until they come to be conclusive representations to which the Ego will refer as to a sort of *legend*[29] of the affective experiences that have been acquired. The *phantastic legend replaces the phantastic enactment*, thereby creating a direct causal nexus. As Aulagnier reminds us, no one preserves the memory of their relationship with the breast but everyone is overcome by a feeling of the same intensity when presented with the image of a baby in its mother's arms as they are in the presence of a newborn infant crying desperately in its feeling of abandonment.

So it is the meeting between historical temporality and desire, as Chabert reiterates, which allows *the origin of the Ego's history to coincide with the origin of the desire that preceded it and brought it into being.* But if this entanglement is to happen, the other must not dispossess the Ego of faith in its memory and in the way it has used memory to interpret its feelings and emotions: only in this way will the Ego be able to reassure itself that the relationship really exists, because in this way its memory becomes complementary to the other's memory, and also guaranteed by it.

Therapeutic potentiality and the difficulty of interpretation

If clinical diagnosis appears difficult, perilous, sometimes hidden and obscure, then treatment is inevitably also complex.

The area where I would like to focus my attention is what I call *therapeutic potentiality*, using this to indicate not only the precarious nature of the therapist's tools in relation to the difficulties of diagnosis and the defences at work, but also the vast resources which this very complexity makes available to treatment.

But if we are to follow Piera Aulagnier along this path we need to pause and reflect on the difficulties that come with reading her ideas, in interpreting them, in making methodological use of them, and applying them in the technique of analytic treatment so we can go beyond the limits imposed by these clinical situations.

The first difficulty in reading Aulagnier has various historical reasons. Like many, perhaps all, French psychoanalysts she was heavily influenced by Lacan's ideas, despite her later break with them. Lacan's thinking is complex even in the best translations, and for all its richness it is characterised by a tendency to particularly dense exposition.

Another reason for the difficulty of reading Aulagnier is the fact that she stands so close to the subject she is studying that she sometimes seems to lose her distance from it. In my view, there are two aspects to this: first, when she talks about the object by talking *as* the object and, secondly, when – as the object – she loses the coherence of her theoretical discourse. I am referring, for example, to her criticism of psychoanalysts who pursue psychiatric diagnoses, calling them entomologists of the psyche; and to the fact that she herself then often goes on to schematise certain – let us say – phenomenological and anamnestic characteristics without submitting her observations, or those of the reader, to the countertransferential work that happens in analysts when they make these distinctions. And this is certainly not because she overlooks the weight of the countertransference – on the contrary, she stresses its inevitable non-neutrality – but because she underlines the autobiographical aspect of the researcher in constructing a theoretical thought. For example, in the work I cited earlier, *L'Apprenti-historien et le maître-sorcier* (1984), she emphasises the fact that every generalisation in psychoanalysis is arbitrary but then indicates two typologies of subjects related to the theoretical discourse that she herself had set up. Her thought thus finds itself in continual movement and compels the reader to move with it, perhaps like the many moves in her own life.

The third and final difficulty derives from the originality of Aulagnier's ideas, which has the weight to construct a metapsychological terminology of her own and endow pre-existing words with her metapsychological valence: originary, pictogram, narcissistic contract, word-bearer, metabolization, identifier-identified, *telescopage*,[30] and so on.

The inevitable additional complication of these ideas is their content: psychosis. And despite the reams of entirely authoritative literature that have been written, there is fortunately a high degree of awareness that psychosis stands on structural and functional terrain that is in part obscure and impervious to treatment, which is why it keeps its power to attract as well as its frightening and sometimes horrifying image.

The complexity of Piera Aulagnier's thought does not make the reading of it any less helpful – and indeed indispensable, in my opinion – but as with any legacy there is a need to make choices and to go through conflicts and even make some transformations.

To back up this claim I would like to go back to a work by Valabrega which adopts a contrasting theoretical position to certain points in Aulagnier's thought.

In an essay published in *Topique* (1, pp. 119–122, 2001) entitled "Les notions de pictogramme et de potentialité psychotique dans l'œuvre de Piera Aulagnier" and to which I briefly referred in the previous section, Jean-Paul Valabrega both highlights the derivation of Aulagnier's thought from that of Freud and to some extent criticises it. This makes it especially interesting for the purposes of my own reflections.

On the *pictogram* Valabrega maintains that it is obviously related to Freud's *mnemic trace*, as Aulagnier herself frequently made clear. His reservation about this refers to the fact that, in his opinion, the term *pictogram* emphasises the graphic and written aspect of the concept which would attribute pre-eminence to the sense of sight at the expense of the others: smell, hearing, touch, and taste. Likewise in the case of *potentiality*, which for Aulagnier is purely psychotic, Valabrega highlights its Freudian derivation, a polymorphously perverse disposition in the child, a disposition to transference and to hysterical conversion, and a predisposition to obsessional neurosis. Here again he expresses reservations and makes more than one criticism.

- He maintains that the field of psychotic potentiality is so vast that it needs a more precise definition.
- He claims that without precise specifications it all risks being founded on hypotheses and conjectures, confirmed by countertransferential projections with theoretical concepts being

constructed retroactively, and one could add, tautologically (for example, if a psychosis develops it means there was a psychotic potentiality).

- He adds that the causes of psychotic potentiality are infinite in number: familial, traumatic, hereditary, acquired – and so its boundaries are fluctuating, a matter of perspective, provisional.

I can readily accept the suggestion that Aulagnier's ideas are related to Freud's but I am less able to share Valabregas's criticisms of either concept.

In the *pictogram*, which refers to a trace as if from a primordial graph, Aulagnier makes very clear the bodily complementarity on which it is constructed, and nothing corporeal belongs to a single sense. So the question is limited to a mere definitional detail, and yet if it is by means of this concept that Aulagnier constructs a hypothesis about the *Originary* (no differently from Freud constructing his two models) it is because this is her most courageously exploratory feature.

On *psychotic potentiality*, I again find myself in agreement about its Freudian derivation, but less convinced about the criticism, since it is absolutely true that clinical journeys are adventures, but it is also true that Aulagnier offers a map with an extraordinary capacity for guiding us, a map that is far from tautological. I entirely agree with Valabrega that nothing much is gained by accepting that once psychosis has become manifest there must have been a prior potentiality for it, though it is never pointless to recognise the fact scientifically and research it: but it is of the utmost benefit to *understand in advance* if a patient who does not seem in any way to present as someone likely to explode into a psychosis does instead have characteristics – the research map indicated by Aulagnier – by which the analyst may be able to defuse this process.

The *theoretical map* should be understood as a functioning in the analyst's mind equivalent to something known but apparently forgotten, which re-emerges as a structuring element like the warp of a Gobelin tapestry before it receives its design.

The aim of these reflections is not merely to celebrate Aulagnier's ideas but to put them into operation: that is, to look for the *non-evidence* about what appears to be evidence of derivatives from the unconscious.

And so we must ask ourselves, what is the new frontier at which Aulagnier's ideas summon us to gather?

Her words provoke readers, disenchant them, compel them to read against all the evidence: essentially, if they have been internalised, they are constantly at work in the analyst's countertransference thanks to the experience they have made possible.

So, what are the difficulties that practising analysts would be required to deal with?

In psychotic potentiality, *a difficulty that does not emerge.*

There is nothing analytic about any move that is inductive or directive, or which merely privileges one aspect selected from those offered by the patient's unconscious, via its derivatives, in the session.

And it is on this point that I would like to dwell further.

Piera Aulagnier's reflections about psychotic potentiality are not just an instrument for reading something that is there, out of sight, to be unearthed but which, once discovered, opens the way to curative treatment. Her reflections put observation into reverse, forcing us to observe that which does not appear. With Green (1993) we could call it a true *work of the negative.*

I would like to suggest a metaphor that came into my mind associatively during a seminar between analysts and literati in which Aulagnier was not the subject under discussion.

On clear nights in late summer, if we make our way to isolated places like those where the psyche can take refuge, we can see, thanks to the lower light pollution (the light of evidence), many of the stars in our galaxy that are otherwise not visible to the naked eye. In a word, we need to make it dark in order to see and – more than Bion's *beam of darkness* – I would say it also means turning off the theoretical light pollution that enriches our countertransference when we are in difficulties, with the risk that we dazzle ourselves and paradoxically darken our path: theoretical and cultural pollutants that, if well-analysed, do not fail to bring out the Oedipal conflictuality that sustains them. But this should perhaps be part of another chapter.

So, to be more precise, I would say that the legacy which Aulagnier's thought bequeaths to clinical practice concerns the unearthing of *primary delusional thinking about origins,*[31] but to do so we need to darken all the defences in analytic listening so that it can emerge through the *darkness of the word.*

The choice of the term is not intended as poetic, although this would certainly do it no harm: it is simply a way to indicate a quality of listening-seeing that, in my view, must be reduced to a cruder, more condensed sensoriality in order to be "heard," as Aulagnier puts it, lowering the other, excessive sensorialities (see also the type of listening proposed by Bollas, 2018[32]).

How then do we make a non-emerging difficulty emerge in clinical work?

Those who have read Aulagnier note that many of the facts given about her patients' history are provided by interviews with their relatives.

This was part of the method used in her programme of research into psychosis in the *Quatrième Groupe*, and we can only be grateful for the wealth of information unearthed and the way Aulagnier elaborated it, although it represents an unusual and wholly unorthodox praxis, at least for those who do not work with psychotics.

Even setting aside the logic of orthodoxy, some qualifications do need to be made. The first concerns the fact that Aulagnier's study falls into the category of research but it must also be remembered that this way of working has shown itself to be indispensable in work with children and adolescents and with psychotic patients because it is not just a search for "*information*" but the analyst's first step towards a possible "*deformation*," which in these cases appears to be missing, or even wiped out: all this within a complex group transference which the analyst can nevertheless elaborate, to some extent more easily than in the initial relationship with a single psychotic patient.

In the opposite case the analyst would risk finding themselves in a bind where the demand is simultaneously made and denied by the group itself, and the analyst would end up being recruited to the role of proxy, a proxy both appointed and repudiated by the psychotic system. The acceptance of the delegated role would risk a further move in the direction of tragically confirming the patient's long-term experience of passivity in relation to the outside world and the Other.

Nevertheless, I would like to reiterate the point that the individual setting is still a valid device of choice for the analytic process; and I would add, paradoxically in the light of what I have just claimed, still more the device of choice in a psychotic situation. So we could picture the two analytic situations as complementary. The individual device therefore remains valid and necessary in a complementary manner to the other, all the more so in situations where we glimpse a *psychotic potentiality*. Because that which is denied or sequestered certainly does not emerge from an interview that digs down, however intensely, into the past, this model of investigation could instead sometimes strengthen the defensive system of concealment or lead to a pseudo-knowledge of the facts, which would not be assimilated and would persist in maintaining its disavowal of the facts as belonging to the subject (stuffing and lining not stitched together, one sliding onto the other without forming or fixing the body of the mattress, to return to Lacan's metaphor of the *quilting point*).

I am drawing these reflections from my experience in regional psychiatric services.

However, even if we take on board Aulagnier's thinking about the origin of psychotic potentiality, this position does not give us any guarantee about the possibility that the factors which predispose to it emerge spontaneously, precisely because they are denied or sequestered, and so it leads us back once again to the fundamental question: how to encourage the possibility of their emergence?

Insofar as this question forms part of an interrogation of the analyst, or rather of their possible "*hearing*," a central question remains: how to use or risk using this *hearing* in the *countertransference*?

Analysts thus find themselves *in the space of non-emergence*.

What is heard is insufficient to predict the possible arrival of the tsunami in the patient's mind. So all that remains are the various forms of silence and the dull sound of words which both refer back to their being enacted, with Donnet, and which Aulagnier would call *pictorial language* and not functions of autonomous thought.

What I mean is that *psychotic potentiality, the primary delusional thinking about origins*, may remain for an incalculable length of time as silent action – that is, an unthought silence – a silence excluded from thought in which the analyst ends up in a sort of boundless swamp with no features or outlines, immersed in a blanket of fog (as I recalled on several occasions in earlier chapters).

Two scenes can often take shape: a manifest one where the patient speaks, with great coherence and sometimes reasoning ability, as well as passion, at least initially; and another more internal to the analyst, their raw countertransferential product, totally confused and befogged, emotionally arid. Here, Aulagnier's word *authenticity* can come to the rescue and help the analyst *hear* that even the passion, or rather the passionate tone, with which the patient may talk about a pseudo-interest, may be borrowed, imitated, not their own, whether or not the analyst is able to recognise it – and this is for various reasons to which we will return.

Two non-analytic references have been of great help to me, and I feel like suggesting them again since the text of this book has certainly not avoided literary and artistic references.

In his 1975 film *Dersu Uzala*, Akira Kurosawa recounts an event in which the two protagonists know in advance the dangers of the journey they must make, but in order to be capable of making it, they rely not only on the tools of geography to map the territory, but on the intuitive knowledge of the indigenous inhabitant who gives his name to the film, and without whose collaboration the journey could have ended in disaster. This example is also cited in Contardi R. et al., in *Fattori terapeutici nei gruppi e nelle istituzioni* [Therapeutic factors in groups and institutions] (1993).

The other reference is to the word made resplendent by the *labor limae* of the *poet troubadour*[33] who can "light up" the heart. Since the luminous word is not a starting point but an achievement, it is preceded by the work of the artisan who has to take off the rust that is covering it, making it opaque, hiding and at the same time corroding it. (In my opinion, this work of gradually removing the rust to make the word of memory shine more brightly recurs in the psychoanalytic process with these patients, and especially in a sort of evolution of their dreams about what must remain hidden because of their *pact*, usually contracted with the mother.)

In clinical practice Piera Aulagnier's ideas lead us to the paradox of regarding as authentic the darkness into which the detail falls – a darkness that includes the passions – and of feeling the need to disambiguate the irrelevant feature placed in the foreground. This need does not have to emerge as a matter of urgency but encounters the analyst as a possibility of emerging, a possibility which may nevertheless fail. It must be stressed that the clinical situation which takes shape is clearly quite different from the search for derivatives of the unconscious based on free associations and the return of the repressed.

It may indeed happen that the approach to the delusional nucleus is stubbornly unwanted, or that it is endlessly attempted but, as in the myth of Sisyphus, everything falls back to the beginning again.

Naturally there are no travel guides to this side of the mountain, apart from the fact that supporting theories are constantly present in the analyst's mind, as well as a continual mediation between the need for care of the patient, which is implicit in the mandate, and a sense of powerlessness; neither is reassuring, but dialectical and conflictual. The presence of these two coordinates is important in preventing the analyst from becoming a proxy. The constant risk of such delegation in fact emerges through repetition in the transference – onto the object more than onto the word – a repetition of the primary passivizing experience: passivizing and, like any repetition, desubjectivating. Giving up delegation and omnipotence, both of which are demanded from and constantly projected onto the analyst with every form of repetition – including silence or weeping – is the basis for a process of subjectivation. It is in fact the basis for an experience that is different from primary experience because it does not re-confirm passivity and, therefore, even if this is all that is achieved, it would be the expression of an enormous potential for transformation.

It should also be remembered that the phantasy scene provided by the patient is not given but becomes a scene through the analyst's interpretation. The analyst faces the further problem of the how and the when. In these cases I feel I should suggest using a sort of *reality-testing of the countertransferential scene* that comes to be created in the analyst's mind, a reality-testing that consists in verifying how capable the patient is at that moment of portraying a scenic representation that is not a defensive construct in the mind of the analyst.

Aulagnier's ideas lay bare the analyst's defences and force him or her to confront their *originary*, even though it is unattainable: this is the only way of getting into contact with what is containing the patient's experience of *primary delusional thinking about origins*.

Using Aulagnier's suggestions we may think, for example, that the patient is living an exported passion, a mirage-passion imposed by the Other. Imitation may be a way of smoothing over this intrusion but also a way of expelling it without filling up the absence.[34]

That which is missing intrudes, and the *intrusion of absence* leads to repetition with the illusory goal of filling or cancelling out the emptiness, as in the case of repeated silence or rhythmic repetitions (see Chapter II).

While this calls on the analyst to verify their potential for coming close to *primary delusional thinking* it is nevertheless easy to imagine that we cannot list its requirements, as if in a readily available and easily consulted promptbook. Let's recall what Valabrega says about psychotic potentiality: an adventurous and exploratory journey.

We can only pay close attention to the revisiting of certain key theoretical concepts such as *transference onto the object and not onto the word* (see the distinction made by André Green, 2004), the *contact transference* proposed by Lina Balestriere (2014), the so-called *negative transference, lateral transferences*, and the working-through of the countertransferential experience that derives from all this, in order to achieve – after repeated attempts – the reanimating of speech in the setting, which also involves dramatizing it (see Chapter II again).

In trying to put together the suggestions made by Jean-Luc Donnet and Emmanuelle Chervet[35] about the *dramatization of speech* in order to create a synthesis between them, I need to say that these authors see it as an intermediate stage towards interpretation that does not concentrate on a single time, but opens out like a fan onto several times and several degrees of expressivity. The affect, appearing again in the dramatization, makes the object present so that it becomes an intermediary of speech.[36] Denied speech (prohibition, the forbidden secret as Aulagnier calls it) returns in action – and in the enacting of the dramatized word – as testimony to the traumatic experience, offering only this possibility of communication. By *presentifying* the object, the analyst may find that the dramatization of speech makes it possible to re-signify what has been denied by the parental figures, promoting an experience of subjectivation which may become the opportunity for coming out of passivity, alienation, and delegation to a proxy, encouraging a transformation and an outright reversal in the transference (certainly by the patient taking hold of lateral transferences and by a capacity in the analyst for making him or herself complementary to them). Indeed, what we see being put into effect in the act are two ways of reading the representation: on the one hand, the representation in relation to the affect and, on the other, the thing-representation being brought into word-representation. The meeting point then becomes the affect that gives the self-perception of the investment's intensity in the present. The purpose of the work of dramatization with the patient is to reduce the tension produced by the affect, so as to make the *presentified investment* possible and allow the perception of thought. (Then again, all psychic activity aimed at an elaborative function employs and consumes free energy.) *The act then becomes legible as the dramatization of a representational necessity*. Dramatization may thus become simply a first phase in a process of interpretation,[37] in which the instinctual impulse is emphasised and this would already transform the emerging point, postponing until later phases the eventual possibility of an interpretative elaboration between anachronistic content and present reality (Chervet, 2017).[38]

If I am asked what clinical and therapeutic value all of this may have, I would have to answer: enormous, and it is from this perspective that I would reread Aulagnier's ideas.

The patient may attain degrees of freedom they had not hoped for, but of course not without risks. They do not in fact come bringing their primary delusional thought, which is secret: secret and denied. They come because they feel unwell and nothing about the link with this delusional structure is evident when they begin their analysis. And care is mandated, which means that *primum non nocere* remains an absolute principle, because *non-care* would do harm and risk the psychotic explosion. And *non-care within care* could reinforce the primary experience, bringing out all the possibilities of re-installing a narcissistic contract with the external and the social, and causing a plunge into psychosis by reinforcing the experience of passivity and desubjectivation.

In my view, thinking about these studies is fundamental for psychoanalytic training.

Non-care may express itself in an infinite number of ways, from an excess of diagnostic assessment to its complete omission with the more or less ideological aim of absolute relativisation: all the ways that can embed themselves in the analyst's defences against their own desire to engage with the psychotic aspects of psychotic potentiality, which also run in both directions.

Untimely interpretations by the analyst have long been criticised, but there has never been much progress beyond an equally persecutory interpretation of their defences. It is much easier than one may think to confuse the patient's enactment in words with a scene resembling a representation that metaphorizes and thus symbolises the trauma. But this scene could be a defensive construction that appears only in the analyst's mind, confusing them about the patient's capacity for dramatization. It is very important for the analyst to take responsibility for this production of their own, but also important that they take care not to export it violently into the clinical situation.

Instead, what I find fundamental for therapeutic purposes – as a potentiality in a state of becoming – is the transgenerational legacy that this type of analytic experience may lay down, precisely because it interrupts the repetition of the identical across several generations thanks to the subjectivating value which the analytic experience is capable of giving.[39]

Patients who, in their analytic treatment, choose ever more consciously to be their own bomb disposal expert, defusing the time-bomb of primary delusional thinking and calling on us as their witnesses – witnesses who are therefore also at risk – are often strongly motivated by the desire to leave a legacy; as if, having made very little investment in their past, they would like to invest heavily in their future: theirs and, above all, their children's. It is a real investment in a state of becoming, which also sometimes draws on the sacredness of hope, a term which, as I have often recalled, is always infused with spirituality, even in secular thought, since it indicates a goal. This differs from what sustains *becoming*, a concept which appears more in shadow because it is less central to the presence of the goal.

I believe that something which the secular thinking of psychoanalysis should not lose sight of in treatment is the fact that this good investment in the future and in the patient's legacy, which entails a separation and hence loss and mourning, is associated with a historicising re-signifying of the past. Otherwise a building would go on being constructed with some pillars missing, which is as bad in its way as not starting out at all. This re-signification is also indispensable for the guarantees that are to be given to the future, a safekeeping to ensure that it remains possible to take responsibility for knowledge of one's origins. Aulagnier suggests that this work of historicising continues to be done until the final session.

Someone might object that every analysis has or may have these characteristics.

We can of course agree to this while also agreeing about the limits of analysability. *Primary delusional thinking* is more at home in these limits than any other feature. This does not make it the "object of a special search" but one that is "re-searched/RE-found," to borrow a definition from both Freud and Winnicott.

In conclusion, I would like to summarise three points of difficulty for the analyst, difficulties concerning the integration of metapsychology with clinical observation:

First, a *deficiency in repression* which we often encounter in these patients. This must be seen as a deficiency of selective symbolisation, perhaps already present in the mother. It may lead patients into an *asymbolic primary signification of their own mother.* (See René Roussillon in *Agonie, clivage et symbolization*, 1999, talking about narcissistic disturbances where the process of symbolisation is missing. The result of this may be that when they are achieved they have the reality of *non-symbolic links* that do not enable access to reality-testing and so leave the subject in a condition of unsayability, which is also the result of their indeterminacy. See also Bastianini T. et al., eds., *L'impronta del trauma. Sui limiti della simbolizzazione* [The imprint of trauma. On the limits of symbolisation], 2009).

In this hypothetical failure to transmit a maternal function, what is transmitted instead is an originary totalising function.

Secondly, there is a *difficulty in contacting this totalising function* in any relationship, and therefore also in the analytic relationship.

And here I cross-refer to Green's (2002) *total and totalising object*: that is, an absolute and absolutizing object produced by a tyrannical agency, an object which crushes the Ego from inside; this is the expression of a deficiency in the phase of primary narcissism, and it creates the difficulty that every object relation is in competition with the transference object.

Thirdly, there is the need to reflect on the fundamental contribution of Piera Aulagnier's ideas about transgenerational transmission and its consequences in the analytic process, a contribution that is fundamental for theoretical-methodological elaboration.

Poets overcome these difficulties better than we do, and so they help us to think:

> My hands are of your colour
> but I shame to wear a heart so white.
>
> William Shakespeare (*Macbeth*, Act II, scene ii)

Notes

1 For further details about the history and development of Piera Aulagnier's thought, see Costis A., "Piera Aulagnier esploratrice instancabile degli abissi originari" [Piera Aulagnier, tireless explorer of the originary abysses] in Cupelloni P. (ed.), *Psicoanaliste. Il piacere di pensare* [Women psychoanalysts: the pleasure of thinking], 2012.

2 Cf. Klein M., *Love, Guilt and Reparation* (1975); *Envy and Gratitude and Other Works* (1975), and in particular the paper "Our Adult World and Its Roots in Infancy."

3 Cf. Bion W., "Development of Schizophrenic Thought" (1967) in *Second Thoughts* (1970). However, it is important to recall that Bion places the emphasis on the non-psychotic functioning inside a psychotic functioning.

4 Cf. Tustin F., "Psychotic elements in the neurotic disorders of children," *Journal of Child Psychotherapy*, 4, pp. 5–18, 1978.

5 I cannot help referring also to Green's *framing structure*.

6 There is an interesting link to a later work, not directly related to the writings of Aulagnier, by Donnet on the three stages of speech: Donnet J.-L., "L'agir de parole" in *Des psychanalystes en séance. Glossaire clinique de psychanalyse contemporaine*, 2016. See also Scarfone D., "L'impassé, l'actualité de l'inconsciente" in *L'actuel en psychanalyse* 5, pp. 1357–1428, 2014.

7 See also a pictorial representation of this which I have found disturbing and significant: George Tooker, Sleepers, 1959, MOMA, New York. https://www.moma.org/collection/works/79548/

8 A return to the undifferentiated occurs in biology when the oncogene is unrepressed and so makes the cell acquire the invasive and destructive totipotentiality that is typical of the carcinogenic cell.

9 Cf. Valabrega's *engram* mentioned later in this chapter. Valabrega questions the term *pictogram* because he regards it as referring solely to the sense of sight. In his opinion, *engram* is therefore more representative and closer to the Freudian *mnemic traces*. "La notion de Pictogramme et de Potentialité-psychotique dans l'oeuvre de Piera Aulagnier," *Topique*, 1, pp. 119–122, 2001.

10 I have chosen to keep the upper case for the Other, both from fidelity to the author's custom and to recall the trace of Lacanian training which shows through in Aulagnier despite her wish for a clear separation. In Lacanian terms the use of the upper case indicates the experience of an unattainable originary otherness, whereas the lower case, the "small object," stands for the residue of the enjoyment achieved by means of the first infantile libidinal experiences, which takes the place of the lost object, an experience which instead corresponds to a total enjoyment.

11 For the concept of representation in Freud see *The Interpretation of Dreams* (1900) and the *Papers on Metapsychology* (1915). In this note I will only repeat what I have said earlier in this book, that the concept of representation in Freud is, like the drive, one of his most heterogenous since it always nevertheless results from a happy encounter between a perceptual quantum which draws as much on sensoriality as on the unconscious, and on an ideational quantum which participates in the secondary process and its more psychically differentiated functions.

12 The purpose of this very condensed clarification is to prevent unhelpful contrasts being made between theories which maintain the indispensability of the Other in making it possible for the *infans* to think: Bion's *rêverie*, for example. There is certainly a diversity of theories but they never contradict each other. The presence of the Other in order to realise the possibility of separateness is fundamental in Aulagnier: her idea about the possibility of preserving an exclusive secret space seems to be a simple snapshot of another developmental moment which by no means rules out the indispensability of the Other, but limits their violent omnipotence which could be harmful to the Ego's development. If anything, it is a theoretical content that fits with the mother's intermittent, necessary, and helpful inattention (to which Winnicott refers), that fleeting non-investment which allows the mother to calibrate and modulate her affective investment of the child. It also fits with that maternal indifference, similar to the analyst's, which Laplanche talks about: this is by no means neglect or rejection but equivalent attention to every content of psychic life. What it means is that if the *infans* has fully passed through the initial phase of autogeneration it is thanks to an encounter with the satisfying and bountiful Other. This positive presence of the Other in the environment fosters the processes of metabolization between states, which is another of Aulagnier's fundamental conceptual contributions. The same clarification could be applied to the definition and identification of "object" based on the recognition of the Ego as its own object in Freud's primary narcissism: but however helpful such an investigation would be in exploiting the profound differences between theories without their necessarily contradicting each other, it could lead us a long way further towards synthesis than we wish to go.

See also the paper given by Chiara Matteini at Florence Centre of Psychoanalysis and published on the centre's website: "Soggetti segreti, destinatari sconosciuti" [Secret subjects, unknown recipients] (CPF, 2017).

13 Distinguishing between loss and absence, Winnicott introduces the psychic space characterised by a *gap*, a *blank* (see *Playing and Reality*, 1971), and gives fantasy (Winnicott's customary spelling) an active role, activating the subject who participates in this creative construction which fills the gap. For Winnicott, fantasy also has the valuable function of enabling a sort of dissociation in the Ego at highly critical moments, which we can rediscover in borderline states, allowing the Ego to be *not there* and thus avoiding the *fear of breakdown* (cf. "Fear of breakdown," *International Revue of Psycho-Analysis*, 1963; see also Winnicott's *Psycho-Analytic Explorations*, 1939–1968; and *Pensiero di Winnicott* (ed. Clement C., 2016).

14 See also Laplanche J., Pontalis J.B. (1985), *Fantasma originario. Fantasmi delle origini. Origini del fantasma* [Originary phantasy. Phantasies of origin. Origins of phantasy], 1991.

15 Freud S., *Leonardo da Vinci and a Memory of His Childhood*, 1910.

16 Cf. Chapter VI and especially Freud's *Leonardo da Vinci and a Memory of His Childhood*, 1910.

17 The term *metabolization,* taken from the biological sphere of molecular theory, refers to a sort of cellular digestion, but it is a very different metaphor in time and scale from that of the digestive tract proposed by Bion, although similarly rooted in reference to organic functioning. The organic aspect – but still more the idea of cellular functioning – metaphorizes the absolute exclusion of these psychic processes from consciousness, those involving the transition from one state to another and also the residue remaining from previous states. What would we ever expect to perceive consciously of what happens during the metabolic activity of cells in the liver, the kidneys, the thyroid, or even the neurons?

18 See *The Ego and the Id* (1923), *On Narcissism: an Introduction* (1914), *Mourning and Melancholia* (1915), *Neurosis and Psychosis* (1924).

19 [Translator's note: the Italian edition of Laplanche's book carries the main title *Il primato dell'altro in psicoanalisi* – The primacy of the other in psychoanalysis – which indicates more clearly the relevance of Laplanche's work to the argument of the present volume.]

20 Aulagnier identifies three *types of identification*:

- *Primary*, the effect of the encounter between *mouth* and *breast*
- *Imaginary*, corresponding to the *mirror stage* and *primary narcissism*
- *Symbolic or the identificatory project*, corresponding to a project of openness to the *identifiers in other people* – the *narcissistic contract* – a process of identification which maintains a potential for conflict.

For Aulagnier the various *psychotic potentialities* are based on the following:
- *Psychotic*, characterised by a crack at the beginning between identifying and identified- *Neurotic*, conflict between the Ego and its ideals- *Polymorphous*, characterised by the pathological conditions of dependency: for example, *alienating* passional relationshipsAulagnier also emphasises the danger of *alienation in identifying with the institution* whenever there is an abandonment of thought or autonomous action in order to eliminate conflict. To which I would add: the alienating process of abandonment that is the basis for any dependency.

21 We may think of fundamentalisms and supremacisms, to name only the forms with an impact on daily life, but I have already recalled in Chapters V and VI the various *-isms* that history has witnessed.

22 As a societal phenomenon, we have to acknowledge the recent denialism about the existence of the pandemic and the use of vaccines. *Supremacisms and Nationalisms* are linked to each other and with *negationisms* and other expressions of *splitting*, and among splittings we must remember all the expressions of *omnipotence* – e.g., the recurrence of "*mega-*". This inevitably gives rise to abuse in a projective and paranoid logic of the fear of being abused, annihilated, and replaced, with fundamentalist consequences. We both see and fear the individual, collective, and political consequences.

23 " 'It seems very pretty,' she said when she had finished it, 'but it's rather hard to understand!' (You see she didn't like to confess, even to herself, that she couldn't make it out at all.) 'Somehow it seems to fill my head with ideas – only I don't exactly know what they are! However, somebody killed something: that's clear, at any rate....' " Carroll L., *Alice's Adventures in Wonderland and Through the Looking-Glass*, pp. 130–131, 1954.

24 It is not hard to rediscover an aspect of Freud's drive theory in this theoretical *décalage*. The *question* is identical to Lacan's: i.e., the mother's constant demand to return to the initial dyadic state. But for Lacan it is a condition with no conclusion, an insuperable lack, while for Aulagnier, as for Freud, it is a question which uses the gap to activate a progressive dialectic that leads to the overcoming of the dyad.

25 The term *mentalised* is used here in a sense very close to the way Michel de M'Uzan uses *mentalisation*. For de M'Uzan, a content is mentalised when the maternal libido has invested it so that the mother can gain access to the child's psyche through his body. And so the child's psyche is first invested by the maternal libido which opens up access to the

subsequent crossings to and fro between body and mind that will be effected by the child.

26 As is also held by Freud and many post-Freudian authors.

27 See again the clinical example of the patient I cited earlier, who left every change to time. It was a tacit compromise, the expression of an unconscious *pact* and signal of a weakened *narcissistic contract*, so as not to take responsibility for a change that she would experience in those moments as catastrophic.

28 *Pointe de capiton* [quilting point]: the concept was introduced as part of *Seminar V* (1957–1958) in an initial lecture given on 6 November 1957 and entitled "The Graph of Desire." The aim of the seminar was indeed to construct a graph and to do this Lacan begins with the relationship between *Signifier S* and *Signified S'* which he illustrates with the metaphor of sewing a mattress. In the 1950s mattresses were still made of wool with a lining, and the stitches that held wool and lining together were called *quilting points.* In the metaphor this point indicates the knot that holds the level of the *Signifiers* together with that of the *Signifieds.* If this does not happen the two planes stay separate as they do in psychosis. In *Seminar III* (1955–1956) on the psychoses Lacan had already said that the relationship between *Signifier* and *Signified* is mobile and tends to be undone in psychosis. Only the points where the *Signifier* intersects with the *Signified* produce effects that have sense. The quilting point therefore indicates the intention of the signification, the intention that mobilises the *Signifier* in the speaker and the listener, an intention to which access can only be gained afterwards in *après-coup.* The quilting point is represented by Lacan with a vector that goes from left to right S-------→S' and another that goes from right to left S←--------S' intersecting with the first at two points.

29 *Legend.* Chabert suggests that it is important to catch the polysemy of the term *légende.* Its polysemic aspect is not as obvious in other languages, despite the shared etymology deriving from the Latin *legendum*, to be read. Here, alongside the meaning *fable* or *fantastical narrative*, there is the sense of an explanatory list appended to a map or a chart.

30 *Telescopage.* A term used by Aulagnier to indicate the slippage of one thing into another, as happens in the movement of a telescope. Indeed, as she says in *The Violence of Interpretation* (1975, p. 169), "on the stage of reality, once that stage has been recognised as an external, separate space, there rises up in a way that is either too intense or too repeated an event that *acts out* a fantasy representation." Here, though the topic is

slightly different, see the point made by Catherine Chabert in the previous section about the link that comes to be created between the relational phases that the child-subject moves towards and its phantasmatic representations, with particular regard to the slippage of the affective resonances.

31 Summed up conceptually, *primary delusional thinking about origins* is the delusional negation of the masculine and the paternal function, together with a prohibition against the possibility of testifying to that function. Primary delusional thinking founded on this relationship between negation and prohibition is the basis of psychotic potentiality and thus proceeds, not repressed but silent, over many generations. Aulagnier devotes almost all the second part of her book *The Violence of Interpretation* (1975) to this piece of theory, starting from *The Economic Problem of Masochism* (1924) on the sources of infantile sexuality, where Freud notes that even the excitation produced by pain and unpleasure provides a component for the sexual drive. Aulagnier considers what happens after a child has witnessed a highly charged external scene; in other words "any event taking place on the external stage that is a source of intense emotion for the psyche, either because it is reminiscent of an experience shared by the actors with the same degree of emotion, or because the interpreter projects this interpretation onto the signs perceived. It will follow that... any representation of external space charged with 'sound and fury', whether it be the sound of mourning, of conflict, of pain, of hate, or of love, is presented, at an early stage of psychical activity, as the equivalent of a primal scene in the strict sense of the term" (p. 194). This is because coitus will not be differentiated from another "sight" that brings the same emotional reaction, and the intensity will be proportional to that which is conferred by the couple and the pleasure they had in displaying it. This will set a defensive disposition in motion, which the child will face by making a "choice" about which of the two parents to choose as an ally against the other. According to Aulagnier, this initial choice is highly idealised and generally falls on the father, both because he represents a powerful ally and in order to avoid the risk of falling back under the deadly, overwhelming spell of the previous relationship with the mother, which would lead the child into a *renunciation of being*. However, this choice does not protect the child from seduction: the idealised is also eroticised, and he in fact allies himself with the one he hopes will seduce him. This will once again lead the child into perceiving himself as a source of conflict every time he perceives himself as desiring, with the result that the

"*desire to fight a desire*" (Aulagnier, p. 197, my italics) will predominate, preventing the Ego from gaining access to a structuring order. But the idealisation will quickly lapse into failure, stirring up hate and rejection of the decay/decadence in which the child's Ego will once again see itself. The intolerability of all this will lead him to preserve the *idealisation of the father, but in the negative*, idealising the mother's suffering. This solution will, however, reveal itself to be fragile, leaving the subject with "that set of features formed by a certain rigidity, a certain mistrust, a certain confidence in one's rights and one's knowledge, that is to say the 'front' that is rigid only in appearance and which allows one to glimpse, behind it, the gulf into which such subjects may fall with each step they take. When the wrong step is taken there will be formed a systematisation of primary delusional thinking; the world will become as paranoiac delusion reshapes it, so that the senselessness of the situation into which his birth projected him may recover some meaning" (Aulagnier, p. 198), a secret inexpressible sense.

32 Conference of the Italian Psychoanalytic Society, Rome, November 2018, *Dalla consultazione alla costruzione della relazione analitica* [From consultation to the construction of the analytic relationship]. See the paper by Christopher Bollas: "Thoughts on the assessment of a person who has just suffered a psychotic decompensation or is having a breakdown." Bollas has proposed terminologies and conceptualisations which, in my view, represent meeting points between different theories. Cf. Bollas, *The Shadow of the Object: Psychoanalysis of the Unthought Known* (1989). In this book he describes the mother, whom he calls the *shadow of the object* (cf. Aulagnier's *spoken shadow*) as a transformative object because, with the ways she cares for him, she induces a *psychophysical idiom*, in an unconscious manner expressed predominantly through the body, a sensory-affective modality, acted before spoken; a way of treating oneself and others that is the fruit of a pre-reflexive, fusional experience. Bollas calls this modality the *unthought known* (cf. Chapter II).

33 Cf. Mocan M., "Un cuore illuminato" [An enlightened heart] in Canettieri P. and Punzi A., eds., *Dai pochi ai molti* [From the few to the many], 2, 1155–1177, 2014.

34 Many authors have considered absence as the basis for thought, beginning with Freud. For Bion absence remains the capacity for thinking symbolically, provided that it is the test and testimony of the emptiness having been filled, a transition without which a risky path opens up in the direction of splitting the mind and schizophrenia. This then

is how emptiness without the Other – i.e., even without the absent Other – may become persecutory and intolerable. And many writers have homed in on this, including Winnicott, who states in "The Fear of Breakdown" (in *Psycho-Analytic Explorations*, pp. 94–95, 1939-1968), "The basis of all learning... is emptiness. But if emptiness was not experienced as such at the beginning, then it turns up as a state that is feared, yet compulsively sought after. The search for personal non-existence can be examined in the same way. It will be found that non-existence here is part of a defence. Personal existence is represented by the projection elements, and the person is making an attempt to project everything that could be personal." Here Winnicott's thought meets Aulagnier's, although in the latter there is an emphasis on the persecutory and intrusive aspect of absence. Other authors, such as André Green, have addressed this point. See also the book by Thuan Trinh Xuan, *La plénitude du vide*, which aims to discover a view of the world in contemporary physics and cosmology that is not so far from or dissimilar to that of traditional Eastern spirituality, where emptiness is lived as a possibility of transformation and change: i.e., life.

35 Cf. Donnet J-L. et al, "Réflexions sur la Dramatisation," *Revue Française de Psychanalyse*, 5, pp. 1529–1534, 2015.

36 There is an inevitable cross-reference to Green's *thirdness*, an intermediate psychic process between the primary and the secondary, and thus also an intermediary of speech. See Green A., "Note sui processi terziari" in *Propedeutica: Metapsicologia rivisitata*, 1995. See also Delourmel C., "Green: rapporti del setting analitico con la funzione metaforizzante della parola e i processi terziari" [Green: relations in the analytic setting with the metaphorizing function of speech and the tertiary processes] in *Rivista di psicoanalisi*, the historical-critical section on *Terzietà* edited by Breccia M., 1, pp. 195–205, 2016, and my introduction to the section "Terzo. Da Lacan a Ogden incontrando Green" [Third. From Lacan to Ogden, by way of Green], 1, pp. 171–174, 2016.

37 Cf. Breccia M., "Le moteur de l'interprétation dans un binôme" [The engine of interpretation in a binomial] in *Revue Française de Psychanalyse*, 81, pp. 1473–1478, 2017.

38 Cf. Chervet E., "Patient et Interprète: *Le domaine intermédiaire*" [Patient and interpreter: the intermediate domain], 77me Congrès des Psychanalystes de Langue Française, *Interpréter*, Paris, 2017.

39 See Chapter II for the theoretical reflections by Kaës and Castoriadis, which widen the subject to include the social and the present.

VIII

IN THE "END": END AS TERMINATION; END AS GOAL

Julie: or the New Héloise

Julie is a character created by Jean-Jacques Rousseau, one around whom an extraordinary epistolary novel revolves. It was first published in France in 1761, initially with the title *Lettres des deux amants* and later as *Julie, ou la nouvelle Héloise*.

I found myself talking about her at a café in Siena, looking out on the Piazza del Campo lit by a warm September sun, with a dear literary friend, an always surprising friend and interlocutor, and it is equally surprising that we never talk either about psychoanalysis or literature, but only about the extraordinary crossovers we engage in when these two cultural frontiers meet each other.

Reading *Julie* some time after that meeting, I made an equally unexpected discovery of the many ways in which that book opens up other, non-literary avenues. The paths were clearly in conflict with each other, but what I associated with this was the fine, subtle, and yet definitely bounded, passage between the two possibilities. This brought me back to the polysemy of the term "end" and to my reflection on the end (as finish, termination) and end (as goal) of existence. That thought had an inevitable impact on my analytic work, becoming deeply entwined with it while also unconsciously drawing its origin from it.

So I wondered if I needed to go back to the extreme difficulty I had experienced some years earlier with my countertransferential work in two important clinical situations. This return would perhaps not be a search for further theoretical underpinning but rather a lateral literary countertransferentiality with a supportive function.

 DOI: 10.4324/9781003747581-9

I have always been convinced, and have often written, that culture, and literature in particular, creates some extraordinary lateral transferences in traumatic situations. Sometimes, if these transferences are properly grasped and welcomed by the analyst, they can become true guides on the path towards a possible representability of the trauma. Why shouldn't this also be true for the analyst's countertransferential work? Particularly so when the clinical situations are so difficult that the internal dimension is not just the *narcissistic curfew* I mentioned earlier in this book, but requires a sort of *elaborative training*, even after a long period of time, with the need for new teachers and new forms of support.

Since this further elaborative element also has "time" and the value of time as a central and demarcating point, I will try to offer a reading which I hope may become a further supportive moment for sharing with my readers.

Jean was a socially successful young man who came to me for analysis because he had been prostrated by his girlfriend's having left him. Jacques was an older man who, after his second wife died, like his first, from cancer, discovered that he too had cancer. And why is he coming to me? His answer is that he needs to "rebuild a testimony." We very soon realise there would in fact be an awful lot to rebuild, but we keep faith with the mandate of rebuilding a testimony.

Despite the melancholic disturbance affecting both men, and especially its self- and hetero-destructive features, and despite an equally traumatic, though profoundly different, origin story, none of this led me to see them as similar. Moreover, their choices of treatment were different: Jean had begun an analysis of three sessions a week, while Jacques opted for two weekly sessions of face-to-face psychoanalytic psychotherapy. The continuity I am highlighting is a different one: the dramatic, intense, and arduous work of countertransference that I had to do with both men in an extraordinary temporal synchronicity, when they both communicated to me that they were in touch with the same end-of-life organisation in parallel to their analytic work with me. A clinical event that was in itself already highly challenging increased its impact enormously by being repeated by two patients, only a few weeks apart and lasting for more or less the same period of time.

This immediately left me asking a great many questions.

Why are they telling me this?

What is the implicit request?

What transferential desire is motivating them?

What was it in me and in my analytic work that had stimulated this, as yet submerged, transferential feature?

How much of all this could be brought into consciousness and possibly made explicit?

What unconscious elements had mobilised that transference of a "request for death?" And what should or could die in order to bring to life, or keep alive, something else?

What role and what meaning did this coincidence and this temporal synchrony have in me, and in my personal and professional life?[1]

While I accepted the need to mourn the likely impossibility of answering most of these questions, I kept repeating them to myself in the illusion that I could find the *end* of the thread in a dynamic continuity that I felt it was essential to guarantee in the analytic work.

The other fundamental element was a continual exercise in countertransferential work, divided between separating and realigning the two clinical situations so as to highlight similarities and differences which might be relevant for both me and the patients. Their age difference was a great help to me in this.

The fact that Jean's first traumatic experiences went back to a little more than two decades previously – traumatic experiences undergone in a prosperous but unhappy family – did indeed create richer and more solid associative elements to add to the traumas of abandonment he had just gone through; but the all-consuming depressive symptom became a kind of Sisyphean boulder: no sooner had he wrestled it to the summit than he let it roll back down again. And this struggle was complicated by the lack of success in his relations with psychiatrists and his consequent lack of faith in a supporting pharmacological therapy.

With Jacques the traumatic experiences of his now distant childhood and adolescence had been no less disturbing but the many experiences of object-recomposition he had sought, and the various life experiences he had undergone with the two principal women in his life, multiplied and confused the qualities of their repetitive features because the traumas had been smoothed out as they accumulated over the decades. Moreover, the perceptual insistence on being face-to-face with me, and his inclination to control the object, sustained the patient in his resistances against diving into a deeper interiority that would be in contact with the earliest traumas.

Both men were living orderly lives and never missed a session, and the things they said to me about their "contact" with the "external organisation" always had a kind of shame about them, as if they were afraid to upset me or do me harm, worrying that their decision might have a real impact on me, and trying to "organise" their possible plan of suicidal action in such a way that this would not happen. I tried to ironize this anxiety about displacing the harm and this externalisation of the organising function which was invalidating their capacity for internal organisation and the function I might be able to fulfil on their behalf.

Nevertheless, at a certain point, using the leverage of the role in which I was constantly being confirmed – that is, to be their "witness" – and the powerlessness caused by the limitations to treatment which resulted from this way of functioning that was being "lateralised" outwards, I simply thought that the only analytically coherent thing I could do was to accept both these mandates. By this I mean I had accepted the role of witness to the thoughts they wanted to leave with me for the future, while their Ego, subjugated to an exchange with a dead object, seemed unable to commit themselves to this new exchange with the analyst. In my countertransferential work I had also accepted that an "external organisation" was busy protecting them to some extent, while I carried on looking after their "internal organisation." I was also trying to lead the analytic work towards the recovery of that inner perception which seemed to me to be a fundamental nucleus on which to precipitate out the other organising elements.

I found it strange, daring, and a bit frightening; and yet at a certain point I reminded myself that this external organisation should in some way be complementary to my work in the countertransference.

There were also some interpretative explanations for my way of proceeding. When the organisation's name was mentioned I no longer silently surrendered to its oppressive representation of death, but emphasised that my task was different, and that it addressed what had not yet been organised internally. And yet what had changed as a result of my countertransferential gains was not so much what I *said* as what I *felt*. I was beginning to think that the "organisation" really could have a liberating, hopeful function, though highly idealised and therefore in the service of tyrannical agencies that squeezed the Ego and pinned it to its limitations and incapacities. So I was trying to free myself from being encircled in this way by dismantling combative ideals and valuing small vital residues that were running along subterranean passageways which had perhaps been excavated before and led to safer ways out, emerging to highlight the fact that my patients' combative plans were idealisations in negative.[2] After this intense and complex transferential-countertransferential work, the climate in sessions changed with both Jean and Jacques. Jean found a psychiatrist whom, for the first time, he did not reject (and perhaps by whom, for the first time, he had not been inwardly rejected), and accepted medication, which also had the important symbolic function of making him acknowledge that he was ill and thus allowed him to "organise" his care on several fronts. In fact he had extended the circle of those who knew about the "external organisation" to include some friends to whom he had confided his intention, and he was able to recognise in his sessions that this communication had a dual *end*: the discovery that there were still people who loved him and the use of their help to challenge his plan to *end* his life, which by this point he no longer wanted to do. I pointed out to him that the two ends had the same desire: a love of life which he had felt was forbidden long before his girlfriend left him.

Jacques, who for many reasons was in a completely different position as regarded his hope for life, began to commit himself to his grandchildren as the real depositories of a testimony, not psychoanalytic but existential, and possible heirs to a rich heritage of ideas and potentialities which he unselfishly felt he wanted to donate to them with no expectation of a return beyond the awareness of having a legacy to donate, to manage properly and "organise." I pointed out to him that, having spent so long letting other people's identities shape his so that he could feel loved, which resulted from a murderous sense of guilt about his two wives (sustained by a psychotic-depressive omnipotence), at last he could leave the field free for a rediscovery of an identity that was anything but impoverished if it required such an important organisational setup to make sure it would not be wasted and dispersed.

The *dignity* proclaimed by the "external organisation" had been re-found, but it was re-located above all in the history of a subject and a person who at last felt autonomous in managing it.

These considerations, which are inevitably also ethical, do not use ethics as an instrument for excluding those who do not share them as part of their own existential journey: they just indicate another direction for engagement by means of psychoanalytic care, and the possibility of making complementary use of what seems alien and unfamiliar, features which, among others, characterised this treatment.

The term "ethics" seems to open a new topic in what I am trying to address, and at the same time it appears profoundly interconnected to the first – the question of choosing life or its opposite – and not separable from it. Therefore, any structural solution, aiming to make a synthesis of this binomial in writing, seems limited and ineffective.

So I am choosing to add only one brief parenthesis about ethics. It is definitely not a parenthesis directed at making a synthesis of that which cannot be joined in a synthesis – because it is a source of continual exploration and new perspectives and openings – but is instead aimed at narrowing the view of ethics to only two criteria.

The first is affective and leads me back to a long exchange I had with a friend, Valeria Egidi Morpurgo,[3] many of whose writings had ethics at their centre, while the second relates to reflections closely linked to my clinical experience.

In the paper she read, "What do we talk about when we talk about ethics in psychoanalysis?" (see note 3), Valeria Egidi recalls the many theories on ethics drawn from the philosophers of the ancient world, such as Plato and Aristotle, and from the moderns, and their various typological groupings. Among these she notes "theories of motives" in which she highlights the utilitarianism aimed at achieving the widest possible well-being while not forgetting the need for a contract which entails the renunciation of a small part of individual liberty for the common good. She also recalls "theories of conflict" among which she includes the whole of Freudianism. According to Egidi – and in this she has my full agreement – Freud has a very pessimistic view of the passage between generations, whether as expressed in the myth of Oedipus or in the birth of civilisation based on parricide, as in *Totem and Taboo* (1912–1913). In *Moses and Monotheism* (1939) the sons also rebel against the father, but Moses introduces an important new element of differentiation from the barbaric horde and unconscious, instinctual parricide: foresight. Moses is a prophet and so he anticipates the collapse of civilisation into barbarism and thus reveals the tragic potential of human relations.

But this *anticipatory temporal breach* prophesied in the Biblical texts is also possible because Moses is not a tyrannical father but a normative one. His law is a law of submission – what law is not? – but it is also a law to which Moses is the first to submit, thereby creating an ethical model to be shared, which naturally cannot help being conflictual since drives and destructiveness do exist: but, as Egidi reminds us, ethics represent the human strength aimed at limiting them. This all happens in a temporality which distances, and by distancing creates thought, since the feeling of guilt is also mitigated in comparison to the deadly act of parricidal murder, and this arc of time may become the expression of a possible working-through. How long and effective the working-through has been is hard to establish by looking at history. *Moses* was published in 1939, the year of Freud's exile, the year after the passing of the racial laws in Italy, the year the Second World War begins, and the year of Freud's death. Just as Moses foresaw the collapse of civilisation into barbarism, so Freud foresees that the antisemitism of the period is the start of an abandonment of limits on the drives, which – as I have found myself saying before – can hardly be said to have been brought to an end by the Second World War, a historic scenario filled with tragic examples of persecution, racism, criminality, and barbarity, and even though it may be a tragic exception, it still leaves open the question: what war is not?

This hypothesis, which is more doubtful than pessimistic, is not intended to contradict the auguries of rebirth and change which have stirred hope in everyone and repaid the sacrifice of so many people who died to make them a reality: my hypothesis aims to create a dialectic with those auguries so that we do not lose sight of present historical developments and fall into easy reassurances by denying the complexity of the current situation.[4] We are witnessing two terrible large-scale wars, or maybe only one – the Third World War which has already started – but as is happening in Ukraine and Gaza, it remains a fight against lies, illusion, and denial, and not just against bombs, missiles, drones, and chemical weapons.

So, going back to ethics, I would like to follow Valeria Egidi in stressing that *ethics is always an ethics of responsibility* (2007, 2019), as Hans Jonas (1979) also calls it, updating and deepening the fundamental distinction which Max Weber drew between the ethics of responsibility (or being aware, responding – i.e., *answering for* the effects of our conduct: *Verantwortung*) and the ethics of conviction (or intention, principles, ultimate and absolute ends: *Gesinnung*). Let's remember that this distinction is considered one of the most heated and controversial points of contention in current politics.[5] For Levinas the *primacy of ethics* corresponds to *being for the other*, having a *responsibility* for the other, and thus being their hostage (*Etique et infini: Dialogues avec Philippe Nemo*, 2006). This is the level on which Valeria Egidi's ideas meet what I have tried to address here, since she is well-aware of the risks and subterranean traps operating in the fabric of ethics and its theories: for example, when it is subjected – to some extent, inevitably – to idealising impulses.

If we accept the hypothesis of a conflictual ethics which, in Freud's terms, limits the instinctual impulses for a collective good or at the very least for a good operating within the widest possible plurality, who becomes the organiser of the conflict, its moderator or mediator, if not the Ego? And it will do this according to the levels of maturity it has achieved,[6] and therefore also according to the defensive systems it has set up. The conflictual dynamic to which Valeria Egidi refers is not so much a conflict between different entities – ethics and morality, for example[7] – but between more or less primitive defensive systems on which the Ego relies as it tries to mediate between idealising superegoic demands and the drives which impel it towards barbaric action. The current wars make all this tragically evident, and in particular the marked disequilibrium of the Ego that is unable to mediate between the demands and the drives; so the result is a vast prevalence of barbaric action, not only in wars, but also in political actions that are so far removed from collective responsibility.

Reaction-formations as positions of idealising goodness, or the sacrificial search for virtuous models, may continually pollute the field with furtively attractive, seductive impulses. Proposing an ethics of pluralism does not overcome this threat and this fragility since any sham unanimity is always fragile.

Talking about seductiveness while trying to outline the nature of ethics seems to be a paradox, if not an aporia, and yet countertransferential experience gives us some confirmation of this. The urge to latch onto an idealised ethical principle is stronger and more devious than it seems because the conflictual tension to which analysts are subjected in their work on the countertransference when they are treating extreme situations is constantly present and very substantial. So it becomes necessary to create more space and time for reflection on these elaborative elements: otherwise defensive systems may predominate in the clinician and allow idealising elements to slip in so subtly and fluidly as to be almost imperceptible. But precisely because they are so easy and reassuring, they are at odds with the tragic complexity of the clinical situation that is currently being lived through. Because is it so difficult to establish the ethical bases for accepting a conflict, no less consideration should be given to the attractiveness of a radical pessimism about the ethical possibilities of humanity.

Referring again to Valeria Egidi, a few years earlier in 2006, in a paper for the *Rivista di Psicoanalisi* entitled "Why does Moses the man still trouble us? Freud, psychoanalysis, and antisemitism," she wrote, "'*Because I was a Jew,*' says Freud in his letter to B'Nai B'Rith, '*I found myself free from many prejudices and prepared to do without agreement with the 'compact majority*'... We could translate this as a capacity for maintaining a critical distance and not blending with the mass. Which also means, among other things, not making absolutes out of authority or the ideal" (*Rivista di Psicoanalisi*, 4, ibidem., pp. 1087–1106).

If we stay with the recognition that an idealising of the negative persisted in Freud in the form of "not having prejudices," we could address Valeria Egidi's question about Moses by interpreting it as the awareness that the individual is civilised not when they stereotypically repeat the models presented to them by civilised society but when they put into action the responsibility for care: care of the individual and society against destructive attacks, which seems largely forgotten in our current society at war.

Perhaps this is the synthesis which best answers to what happened in the two analytic processes I have described here, where the threats to progress were both an ideal of salvation, conflictually present in the analyst's countertransference, and society's offer to the patients of an easier solution to their solitary conflicts, but also a solution which clearly did not answer to their subjectivity and was therefore used as a stereotype that could be idealised.

Evading these threats probably aided the process of recovering the subjectivity that had been crushed by suffering.

Viviane Chetrit-Vatine[8] talks about an analytic situation similar to the "matricial space," referring to Laplanche, who reminds us how the transference may be prompted by the analyst and describes the "matricial space" as the rediscovery in analysis of the *originary* relationship. "And what the analyst offers... is the rediscovery of the primary relationship" ("Du transfert, sa provocation par l'analyste" in *Le Primat de l'autre en psychanalyse* [The primacy of the other in psychoanalysis], 1992, p. 430). And the question Laplanche imagines the infant asking himself is: "What does the other person want when she feeds me with her breast, and why does she want to do it?" The question is immediately repeated in the analytic relationship: "What does the analyst want? Why has s/he chosen to be an analyst? Why is s/he agreeing to see me?" ("Du transfert, sa provocation par l'analyste" in *Le Primat de l'autre en psychanalyse* [The primacy of the other in psychoanalysis], 1992, p. 430).[9]

The question is not persecutory but opens the way to the *enigmatic.* The transference is *transference of the enigma.* Patient and analyst thus find themselves face to face with the enigma. Hence the term *transference of the matricial space.* How to transform this enigma into a responsible awareness is a fundamental question in every analysis. According to Chetrit-Vatine this happens in the analytic process because the analyst is being charged with effecting the transition from an *enigmatic message* to an "*enigm-ethical message*" by means of what she paradoxically calls *ethical seduction,* because the transference – which, as we know, is libidinally invested – finds an ethical extension with the analyst in the present time.

For Scarfone ("*L'impassé, l'actualité de l'inconscient,*" 2014) the enigma leaves a residue of something opaque which nevertheless survives with a new spirit, mutated by psychical working-through, and becomes a sort of incitement to a word that wants to be spoken as the expression and manifestation of an ethical subject.

It is very interesting indeed to think again about what these two authors have written, but it is as well to remember that we are never spared conflict – no libidinal investment is – or the possible influences of the Superego. In fact no analyst is exempt from the risk of being seduced by an ethic infused with the influences of this internal agency, which idealises to the point of tyranny and turns reassurance into a conformist stereotype.

It was while working my way through these reflections, poised on a knife-edge, as it were, that I was gripped by the discovery of Rousseau's novel *Julie: or the New Héloise,* an experience that was also demanding and complex, especially in requiring me to confront the prejudices which it unexpectedly brought to the surface. One prejudiced assumption was to see the author as a deluded proponent of the virtuous man who, by opting for the universal, trivialises and eliminates conflict, at the high price of sacrificing his characters' individual subjectivity. Obviously Rousseau knew nothing about the theories of conflicting drives, but as I read his book I actually found that he is a great expert on them *ante litteram*; he does not by any means trivialise conflict, but on the contrary seems to keep it alive throughout his novel, though he gives it an illusory resolution. For this reason I found myself plunging enthusiastically into the text and into the introduction by Elena Pulcini.[10]

The title, alluding to the well-known amorous correspondence between Heloise and her tutor Abelard (*Abelard and Heloise. Letters, 1132–1135*) which took place five centuries earlier, announces that the novel is epistolary, a literary form which is perhaps better suited than any other to keeping conflict alive: conflict between the passions and respectable, virtuous conjugal love, and thus not characteristic of the Enlightenment. In fact, Rousseau succeeds in tapping the roots of his characters' Egos, revealing their most representative parts (on this, see Chapter VI on the features of autobiography).

A noblewoman, Julie d'Etange, falls in love with her tutor Saint-Preux, a man of great inner worth but from a lower social class, who is therefore absolutely unacceptable to Julie's family. Instead they want her to accept the marriage proposal of de Wolmar, a wealthy man who in their eyes represents the security of a solid marital bond.

The relationship between Julie and Saint-Preux remains hidden for years, but in the end it is broken off by Julie herself to prevent distress to her parents: and then, after her mother's death, she marries de Wolmar. During the wedding celebrations she convinces herself that it is impossible to continue a relationship with her lover and instead suggests that they maintain a tender friendship. In his despair and disappointment Saint-Preux goes away to sea and only returns many years later. And this concludes the first of the three parts. Julie has accepted her condition as wife and mother and is convinced she is not doing so out of banal submission or from some illusory advantage to be gained by fulfilling the conventional ideal role of wife and mother.

And yet it is evident in all this that the historical-social influences of the time remain clearly apparent below the surface of the writing. This search for an identity, so difficult and of course so conflictually contested because constantly threatened by the risk of becoming embroiled in passions, nevertheless struggles to emerge while contradictions and traps lurk in every corner.

The next three parts of the book are pictures of marital happiness.

When Saint-Preux returns from his travels, de Wolmar presents him, and his own wife, with a model family that reflects the Enlightenment ideal of a society in which a plurality of thoughts and opinions can be freely expressed, and asks him to act as tutor to his two sons. Saint-Preux seems to try and conform to this request, and also to Julie's model of happiness, a model which may allow them to move on from the urges of the past and their attendant dangers while nevertheless keeping the memories alive. However, something gets blocked here because the memory is so alive that it can probably no longer be considered a memory: i.e., a transformation of the experience in the present. And it is precisely this re-actualising of the past which in fact reveals certain flaws, such as a dream interpreted by Saint-Preux as a premonition, or the impossibility – as Saint-Preux sees it – of marrying Julie's widowed cousin Claire, a marriage suggested to him by Julie herself. However, in the end it is Julie who is most subjected to the pressure of the conflict since she experiences another reality which, though characterised by a different feeling, is nevertheless a conjugal reality.

The sixth and final part in fact ends tragically.

During a walk by the lake, Julie's son Marcellin is in danger of drowning and Julie, after throwing herself into the freezing water to save him, becomes ill and confesses on the point of death that she never stopped loving Saint-Preux. She comforts herself with the thought that in the afterlife she will be able to live more freely with her love for him.

Here too various interpretative scenarios are opened up: passivity towards conformism and hypocrisy; a lost illusion about a virtue that was actually only a superegoic repression of the passions; the dramatic reliance on death to achieve freedom; and more besides.

The point I would like to dwell on is the feeling of love being liberated by death, and of liberation by death generally, my aim being to dismantle, at least partly, some facile interpretative scenarios.

It is certainly a rebellion by Jean-Jacques Rousseau against hypocrisy and conformism, and he clearly had no theoretical tools for highlighting the superegoic trap that lies in wait for every ideal, although he never offers a naïve faith in an ideal.

Nevertheless, there is something in the way he sets out his ideas that goes "beyond" this. The "imaginary objects," as he calls them, objects which are perhaps the same ones that formed his characters and shaped the epistolary layout of the novel he calls a "*douce et folle rêverie*" (*Confessions*, 1782, Book IX), also correspond to some aspects of his autobiography, as Elena Pulcini points out in her introduction to the Italian translation (see Chapter VI). In Rousseau's life a series of disappointments overlap with each other, among them his marriage to Thérèse. He meets and gets to know Sophie at the very time he is bringing the character of Julie to life. Social disappointment is added to that of his marriage, causing him to live in a state of deep loneliness.

And yet, in my opinion, the novel overturns its inevitable autobiographical source once again to advance into the future, albeit a partly imaginary one, perhaps in the hope that the author's life might follow suit. In this way, the imaginary seems to compensate for the disappointment of reality, and it sometimes seems as if Freud is speaking, but Rousseau is less clear than Freud about the risk of a failed outcome for his imaginary constructions, as he also is about the entangled dynamics between life and death instincts which accompany them. Yet again it seems as if these theoretical structures, which came two centuries after Rousseau, had underpinned his philosophical and literary thinking and his reflections about existence.

The concept of *doubleness* is very much in Rousseau's mind and is a recurring element in his epistolary novel (a double preface; a doubling between his life and that of his characters; the duality of his imagination paralleling his life; and the mirror image of Narcissus – about whom he had written a play in 1752: *Narcisse, ou l'amant de lui-même*). In fact, as Pulcini notes, he had dual intentions: to write not only a love story but a moral one with love and friendship almost indistinguishably interwoven, since in fact Julie attains virtue specifically through love. On the many levels of conflict suggested by the recurring presence of the double, we could also read, with a metapsychological eye, the conflict between desire and prohibition, foundational elements in the construction of fantasy, which dominates Rousseau's imagination.

This is the representational possibility that leads the author to a choice about the solution for his novel: the choice between a tragic solution, which Rousseau had intended in a first draft, and a conflictual solution, which becomes the definitive choice. As indicated in Pulcini's introduction, Rousseau had initially thought in terms of a four-part novel[11] to end with the death of both lovers, whereas the novel he actually wrote and published a year later rejected that solution in favour of the conflictual one.

The excessive rigidity of every rule leads inevitably to transgression, and it is against this rigidity that Rousseau seems to be fighting. Julie's "Virtue" is complex and so, of course, conflictual: it has no predominantly sexual connotation, nor is it a severe moral prohibition of a superegoically severe kind; it is not even a stoical repression. Perhaps Rousseau is thinking more of a *counterbalancing between the passions.* In fact, it is the story of Julie's slow, laborious progress towards the discovery/rediscovery of her own identity, and I feel I should add that the search for an internal cohesiveness intrinsic to it is complicated by the inevitable multiplicity of identitary aspects (cf. Chapter IV).

The immediacy of the epistolary style makes it easier to catch the elaboration of this intense internal work through the constant instinctual threats to which it is subjected, and in this respect it is different from the correspondence between Heloise and Abelard. It is this difference which makes Julie the new Heloise.

For Rousseau *le veritable amour* is the consolation of a friendship that is care for the other person, but also becomes a guarantee of not losing oneself through a self/hetero-destructive passion.

In all this there remains the persistent illusion of achieving a reality without conflicts which "purifies" the passion through a sort of "reversal",[12] but also has faith in a feminine that thus appears totipotent and therefore inevitably threatening. "I pride myself on the friendship that joins us as a reversal without example," Julie will say to Saint-Preux (letter 6, Part VI, p. 545).

In the novel, the liberation of/from feeling by death is rendered as a ruinous event. So it is not tragic other than in the drama of its style and the texture of the story, and thus it maintains the bases between elements in opposition and contrast, conflictual bases which support the whole work while also representing the way out, albeit a precarious one, from the conflict between illusion and reality.

Going back to Saint-Preux's "premonition" in a dream, which is found in a letter he writes to Julie's cousin Claire (Part V, letter 9), it centres on a mother's deathbed scene, tearfully witnessed by her daughter. The dreamer associates this with a memory of Julie telling him about her own mother's death, and the association becomes a sort of oneiric hallucination in which the character becomes Julie: "I saw Julie in her place" (p. 505). In the dream Julie asks her mother to take back the gift of having brought her into the world, but Julie is covered by a veil which Saint-Preux, in a sort of somnambulism, tries to lift by waking himself up. The dream is repeated three times and as soon as he wakes he asks his friend Edward for help. The practical Edward tries to bring him back to reality by taking him to the Wolmar house. The exposure to reality seems to reactivate the virtuous circle in which Saint-Preux constantly tries to position himself, recognising that the veil was projected,[13] not towards the outside, but into him: "that veil that long clouded my reason" (p. 507). Saint-Preux's dream becomes a phantasy-structure passing through a real which, even if it has perhaps not been achieved as a result of reality-testing by the protagonist, acts as a brake on his state of almost hallucinatory disorientation on waking, and encourages this *retour* to a psychic function: phantasy. In fact, as is well-known, phantasy is an expression of both desire and prohibition,[14] and it brings the subject into play as builder and spectator of the scene, and often its protagonist too. I find that this *retour* must be understand as antithetical to the chasm of tragedy, where the real imposes itself in its tragic dimension with no chance of appeal to any alternative psychic solution that would enable a return. The same thing seems to happen in the final situation where Julie dies, but the suicide of the two lovers that appeared in the first version of the novel no longer features. Here too there is an anxiety which anticipates the dramatic scene, and then everything happens with everyday naturalness: a little boy disobeys his mother, runs, and slips into the lake; his mother throws herself in to save him while the governess and the others are motionless, paralysed. Having rescued the boy and brought him ashore, the mother is absorbed in drying and reviving him, and only then thinks of herself, at the cost of her life.

The fact that death is liberating for Julie should not prompt us to facile interpretations about her unconscious impulses, even when, in a letter sent to Saint-Preux immediately before the event, she entrusts the upbringing of her children to him and hints at death: particularly so because she makes no attempt to acknowledge her own ambivalence.

Julie is right to think it is indeed only death that brings relief from conflict: the key question to be grasped is whether or not the psyche has functioned appropriately to make conflict tolerable during life.

The fatal outcome of the incident is communicated to Saint-Preux in two letters: one from the governess, the other from Julie's cousin Claire. Even the governess's letter, like the phantasy scene mentioned earlier, has the literary structure of a theatrical *pièce*: "Oh

Monsieur! Oh my benefactor! What tidings have they instructed me to send you?... Madame!... my poor mistress... Oh God..." (p. 576) and concludes, "Oh my dear Monsieur, may the good Lord sustain you in this trial.... Farewell... the doctor is leaving the room. I run to meet him... if he gives us some hope for the better, I will add a word to that effect. If I say nothing...." (p. 577).

The exclamations and suspenseful ellipses, the description of movement – almost a vocal communication via WhatsApp – indicate uproar, hope, and the gloomy prognosis, but not tragedy. The death is not described: death is not even named, only dramatically hinted at – "If I say nothing...." And even though Claire's letter gives a few more lines of explanation, it too makes no mention of death. "You will never see her again... the veil... Julie is no.... She has written to you...." (p. 577).

I have also found it interesting to seek out the changes made by the author to the tragic resolution of the unpublished edition, which originally concluded in four parts. Part IV of the definitive edition is redolent of a troubled transition, but also of the whole impulse towards escape from a tragic denouement.

Without embarking on a digression about tragedy, of which no summary would be sufficient, Aristotle's definition in the *Poetics* seems especially apt at anticipating what Rousseau is trying to create and I am trying to interpret in his novel, and the parallels with clinical work that it has prompted me to identify. Aristotle defines tragedy as

> the imitation (μιμησις) of an action that is serious, complete, and of a certain magnitude; in language embellished with each kind of artistic ornament, the several kinds being found in separate parts of the play; in the form of action, not of narrative.... Character is that which reveals moral purpose, showing what kind of things a man chooses or avoids. Speeches, therefore, which do not make this manifest, or in which the speaker does not choose or avoid anything whatever, are not expressive of character. Thought, on the other hand, is found where something is proved to be or not to be, or a general maxim is enunciated.
>
> ("Definition of tragedy" in *Poetics*, VI, 4th century BCE)

It is this feature, the difference between acting and narrating the scene, together with the specific quality of deferred time, that I find central to the differentiation of tragedy from whatever lies outside it.

And so, returning to the conclusion of the Part IV in the later modified and published text, we find a letter written by Saint-Preux to Edward, a figure with whom he has a controversial relationship throughout the novel. In this letter Saint-Preux tells Edward about an excursion on the lake with Julie (the lake again: perhaps an anticipation of the ending in Rousseau's mind), accompanied by boatmen and servants. After two hours' fishing, during which Julie commands that the fish should be put back in the water, they row further out on the lake. The expression used by Saint-Preux is "begun to *stroke*," which is explained in a note as "a term used by boatmen on Lake Geneva. It means to handle the oar that controls the others" (p. 422). Soon the waves become "awesome," making it hard to return, and it is an immense struggle to avoid the rocks in the middle of the lake, during which Julie exclaims, "O my children, must I never see you again?" (p. 423). Finally, with a great effort, they make it to the shore and, after a pause, they walk up to a rocky outcrop overlooking the lake, which had been the place for their amorous encounters, and once again – as on the water – the passionate impulse prevails. The wave of memories floods over Saint-Preux who, for a moment, seems totally unable to govern them, as had happened in the past when, on a similar occasion, he had been very strongly tempted to seize Julie and plunge with her into the waves. On that occasion, he recalls, he let go of Julie's hand and "there my keen agitations began to take another course" (p. 428). He acknowledges to his friend Edward that on that day he had experienced the strongest emotions of his life, but attributes the victory to Julie in the great battle with those emotions, and the letter ends with the question, "how did I manage to remain that far from her?" (p. 428).

All of Rousseau's internal transformative steps appear in this letter, operating through the character of Saint-Preux to avoid the tragedy which twice seems to present itself as a temptation, as if the author had wished to leave an autobiographical testament of his inner conflict about what conclusion to choose for his novel's ending. The tendency to action is continually replaced by story-telling or recollection, a representation of conflict, enabling Saint-Preux with difficulty to escape the urge to enact it under the illusion of annulling it. The denouement brings triumph over the urge, although the Ego is not given the merit for this: instead the author seems to abdicate in favour of an ideal and superegoic image projected onto the beloved woman.

Reading Rousseau led me to re-signify in *après-coup* the intense clinical experience I described earlier, but also to discover parts of me that had certainly operated beneath the surface to ensure an evolution that was not tragic, although it had done so in synergy, and perhaps in synchrony, with what I had been able to bring to light in my work on the countertransference.

Much of what I have read and written has taken the form of connectors whose greater explicative intensity I am now in a position to identify, and I know they have in any case been present and re-presented in me.

There is a still an open enigma about the mind's different times, a multiplicity that André Green wrote about with careful attention while stressing that many deferred times may be synchronous with each other. And what better than writing and literature to bear witness to all this, although all art forms have it in them, as *Le Mystère Picasso* reminds us? (See Chapter VI.)

In *L'avventura del personaggio* [The adventure of the character] (2004), Arrigo Stara, a man of letters and another dear friend who has left us, notes that human beings read to ask questions: and truer words are hard to find.

Which leads me to Atahualpa, the last leader of the Incas, who says he cannot hear or understand what the words on the little white sheets are telling the white man who is consulting them.[15]

> Staggering, he walked down the long narrow street toward where the darkness converged, where the night pressed in upon him, where nothing waited for him, where he was, at last, alone.
>
> (John Williams, *Nothing but the Night*, 1948)

Notes

1 This concept of temporal synchrony is described by Green in *Le Temps éclaté* (2000) and picked up again in *Key Ideas for a Contemporary Psychoanalysis* (2002), preserving the semantic halo offered by the first, originating conceptualisation by Jung as synchronicity. For Jung these are coincidences that involve two more people who share the same experience in a temporal synchronism that may even be repeated over

time, as for example in the anecdote of the plum-pudding reported by Camille Flammarion.
https://subsublibrarian.com/2022/06/30/monsieur-de-fortgibu-and-the-plum-pudding/

In essence, synchronicity for Jung serves as an *acausal connecting principle*. For the theoretical ideas which he derives from this, see Jung C.G., *Synchronicity* (1952).

2 In the *Canticle of the Creatures* St. Francis of Assisi sings about *Sister Death* last, not only to indicate that death comes last, but also because this is perhaps the most difficult praise to sing.

3 Many of Valeria Egidi's reflections, which were the subject of our dialogues and debates, are also recorded in a small e-book which collects the contributions to a Scientific Training Day in Rome, 12–13 October 2019, on "*Etica, Identità, Qualità*," an event which took place barely two weeks before she left us. These reflections of hers represent a lively contribution to her huge, lifetime's body of thought about ethics, Judaism, psychoanalysis, collective traumas, and advancing age: her contribution remained lively until her final days, and still lives in us, not only in our memories but in what she wrote.

4 For Freud, as we know, conflict is structural, and every psychic structure is extended beyond the individual since it is characterised by an intrinsic becoming: for this reason it too is always conflictual. Psychic extension could be seen in terms of passing from a structural conflict to a structure that is always conflictual.

5 See Weber, 1919, "The Profession and Vocation of Politics" in *The Vocation Lectures*, 2004.

6 See the many unethical and irresponsible behaviours during the explosion of the coronavirus: the information withheld by politicians of every nationality for political and/or economic interests; the difficulty scientists had in saying "we don't know" when interviewed on media platforms; the way some politicians pounced like jackals on this or that governmental failure; the abandonment of the weakest in society, an abandonment challenged in words but often, if not always, unchallenged in action; the inconsiderate, dismissive attitude of some groups who could not accept restrictions; or the lack of individual responsibility, delegating everything to institutional decrees; and many, many more. However, we must also remember the ethical behaviour of many health workers and "ordinary" people who simply focused on care and respect, both of themselves and others.

7 Despite their equivalent etymology ("moral" being derived from the Latin *mos*, which is equivalent to *ethos* in Greek) there are linguistic differences

that do not allow ethics and morality to be treated as synonyms. *Mos* still indicates a codified system of recognised behaviours in a community, and so, by "moral," we mean behaviour that can be assessed in terms of value and conformity. Raphael's painting The *School of Athens* distils these differences and their interweaving: Plato is represented with a finger pointing to the world of the Ideas, while Aristotle is holding the Nicomachean Ethics to show that no ethics can be separated from experience. www.arte.it/foto/600x450/5c/64921-RAFFAELLO_-_Scuola_di_Atene_-_Stanza_della_Segnatura_OSRAM.jpg

While ethics, as a science, has claims to universality, morality necessarily presents itself as transitory since it concerns a behaviour which is recognised by a community and may therefore be modified. Descartes is the emblem of the transitory nature of morality with his idea that mankind must give themselves a "provisional morality" while they await a better formulated ethics.

I would say that the essential difference lies in the fact that morality is not the real subject of philosophical, sociological, scientific, and cultural research, whereas ethics is. Indeed, ethics cannot be limited to describing and rationally grouping together a series of value-elements but, while immersing itself in the historical reality which offers those elements, must try to interpret them on theoretical levels that are always under construction.

For the reasons which I have tried to set out very briefly here, ethics and morality can often find themselves in conflict.

8 Cf. Chetrit-Vatine V., "La personne de l'analyste ou un espace matriciel pour M. E." in *Revue Française de Psychanalyse*, pp. 1751–1757, 2004–2005. See also Chetrit-Vatine V., *La séduction étique de la situation analytique: aux origines féminines /maternelles de la responsabilité pour l'autre*, 2012. Also Chetrit-Vatine V., "Toucher à la dimension d'infinité quand le sexuel est tout autant au rendez-vous" in *Revue Française de Psychanalyse*, pp. 1507–1512, 2018. See also Chapter V for reference to the 80th Congrès de Psychanalystes de Langues Française, held online 13–16 May 2021, *Espace psychique, lieux, inscriptions*, where she collaborated with Eva Weil on the report "Espace psychique, lieu analytique, makom."

9 My translation.

10 The introduction to the Italian edition *Giulia o la nuova Eloisa* (1992) is by Elena Pulcini, a social philosopher at the University of Florence, and is entitled "J-J Rousseau: L'Immaginario e la Morale."

11 From the introduction to the Italian text of *Julie* cited earlier: "the first edition of *Julie: ou la Nouvelle Héloïse* was published by Ray,

Amsterdam, 1761. On the novel's editorial history… cf. Guyon, *Note sur l'établissement du texte* OCII, p LXXI–LXXIX."

12 In the original text the term translated as "reversal" is *retour*, which maintains the ambivalence of *veritable amour* as a whole since it also indicates a return to a *quo ante*.

13 Cf. *The Schreber Case* (1910). In this case study, talking about projection, Freud makes a correction which he left visible rather than removing the original version from the published text. He had stated that *internal perception*, which is reduced in projection, was *repressed* and he corrects this in relation to paranoia, saying that it is in fact *abolished*. I have always found this literary practice of Freud's interesting and curious, leaving the corrections in the text, as can easily be found in many notes. The correction is in fact an addition rather than a substitution: an invitation to a multiple writing and rewriting. This certainly has a historical and literary value, and testifies to a scientific way of proceeding but, in my view, also keeps several solutions open. Addition seems aimed at emphasising the recurrent idea in Freud of a continuum between the pathologies and between pathology and normality. (cf. Chapter VII).

14 Cf. Laplanche and Pontalis, *Fantasme originaire. Fantasmes des origines. Origines du fantasme*, 1985.

15 An episode described by historians and men of letters such as Waldemar Espinoza, but also by Felipe Guamán Poma de Ayala, a historian from the late sixteenth and early seventeenth century, who recounts the meeting between Atahualpa and Francisco Pizarro's envoy Fra Vincente de Valverde at Cajamarca, which is now in Peru: Biblioteca Nacional Colección, Madrid, *Nuevo episodio de la Crónica y Buen Gobierno-Atahualpa preso en Cajamarca*, 1615.

The episode takes place immediately after the Inca civil war, from which Atahualpa's army emerged victorious, and the concomitant arrival of the Spaniards in Peru. Here Atahualpa failed to understand the strategy by which the Spaniards arrived in Camajarca in November 1532. Their commander, Pizarro, sent Fra Vincente de Valverde to parley with the Inca leader, which he did in the stereotyped manner expressed by the *Requerimiento*, in which the Spaniards, brandished the Bible as they demanded the submission of the indigenous peoples.

IX
CONCLUSIONS

Thinking about the way Rousseau decided to conclude his novel, a task he found so challenging that he wrote the ending twice, I wondered about how I would conclude this book that is certainly not a novel.

Every ending is conflictual in more than one respect.

On the one hand there is a desire to leave endings to the reader, so as to avoid the narcissistic wound of abandoning a text which has been a life companion for several years; and on the other hand there is the need to separate oneself from it for the same reason, so that it can be allowed its own life.

How does one conclude a volume entitled *Counter-Time*?

Time does not conclude: it takes hold of us, cuts across us, and we have always wondered about our being-in-transformation and what is transformed *in time*.

When we are in contact with Nature it makes us feel the infinite transience of our existence as well as the force that pushes life forwards, and on which everyone builds their representation in phantasy of their own subjectivity.

It is also true that when a book is ended, new paths open up in the writer's mind, and we can make some hypotheses about their origin:

- Avoidance of mourning by premature displacement onto other objects?

DOI: 10.4324/9781003747581-10

- Inexhaustibility of viewpoints aiming at an impossible perfection that might embrace them all?
- Evidence of neglected states of conflict?

Perhaps more of this; perhaps none of it.

It is possible, for example, simply to think about giving space for other perspectives: a way of silencing ourselves as individual subjects to make room for a more harmonious interplay between past and future.

While engaged in this concluding self-questioning I came across a text written by a colleague and friend, Anne Denis, after the death of her husband Jean Capiaux, which reappears in her contribution to a jointly authored paper entitled "Anamorphoses et Atemporalité dans l'oeuvre de Proust" published in the *Revue Française de Psychosomatique* (55, pp. 111–134, 2019).

In this essay the authors note that the end of Proust's *Time Regained*, the seventh and final volume of *A la Recherche*, was in fact written at the same time as the beginning of the whole sequence, as Proust wrote to Mme Straus in 1909, "je viens de commencer – et de finir – tout un long livre"[1] (*Correspondance de Marcel Proust*, p. 163). Looking back in this volume, Proust casts a retrospective light over the entire work (a *Nachträglichkeit* of the kind dear to Freud?), giving new meaning to what has been narrated. The authors write,

> The whole work disguises a time that does not exist (as both Beckett and Rousseau had also noted) where the non-place had triggered the immense work of *A la Recherche*: but when a time has been lost, it is not rediscovered even by a work thousands of pages long. What can be described, however, in minute detail and with "probity," are the consequences of this lack, and one may become the curator/carer – *le clinicien* – of one's own atemporality. *This atemporality is to be distinguished from the timelessness of the unconscious.*[2] It is the atemporality of a lost time, one that did not happen and was not introjected, but belongs to a defective primary narcissism. Time in Proust – or Kant – does not refer to a linear time but to that *intimate experience of time*[3] that Valéry called "*la sensation de ma vie*" which silently accompanies the various aspects of a human existence. The proverb "whoever has time has life" succinctly sums up the enigma of time that has so occupied the philosophers.[4]
>
> (2019, p. 112)

And, as a summing up of their studies, they continue with a backward glance at some philosophical ideas about time:

- "Time as the sensation of one's own life (Valéry)
- as a way of representing oneself (Kant)
- as a condition of all internal phenomena (Kant)
- as natural knowledge without words (Pascal)
- as implicit knowledge which vanishes when one tries to explain it (St Augustine)" (ibidem., p.112).

Which leads them to a question: "Will the philosophers' time turn out to be in tune with the psychoanalytic concept... of an original temporality of the subject who is built up from representations of the drives (the sonic rhythms)?" (ibidem.).[5]

This remarkable study seems to open the way to a further treatment, to another book, one on *originary trauma*, the representations of the sonic, and the various temporalities entailed in all this, along with further immersion in literary, poetic, and philosophical material. My citing it testifies to a desire for a "further" with no end.

But writing-time must come to an end if it is to open itself up to the time of the other, the reader's time, and their returns.

In this book I have tried to document, testify to, and continue to think about how psychoanalysis can engage with that psychic suffering which tries to stop time in order to give the self an unconscious chance of survival.

I have tried to do this by means of the many individual and social, historical, and literary forms that are part of a heritage on which we can all draw, though in a variety of ways and with distinctive characteristics. I have also tried to rediscover in history and literature, as well as in clinical practice, those traces of symbolic possibilities which suffering has submerged, so as to restore them to an inevitably conflictual vitality. On the other hand, the shadow zones and gaps in perception, present as a pervasive rumbling, are an inalienable part of human experience, and all it takes are a pandemic and wars to confirm this. While the pervasive rumbling of the pandemic may now seem far away, we have tragically entered a global war so close to all of us that its pervasive rumbling is no persecutory hallucination: it comes into our homes and our minds every day. This tyrannical insolence, which most of us have never wanted, is a part of our life, to be lived even if never chosen; but history teaches us that the choice of war always goes in this way. Not to mention the pervasive rumbling of floods, avalanches, and fires in entire regions of the earth. So, above all, we have to re-calibrate our psychic defensive order, both individual and collective, to live our present time, mindful of our historical time, and looking forward to a future good enough to leave as a legacy.

Freud wrote that the Ego is always behindhand, always later than the instinctual impulse that precedes it, which complicates its understanding of reality. This wise and modulating view – unlike the assorted omnipotences of "always coming first" and the various moving goalposts imposed by narcissistic slaveries – does not wholly answer to the temporal expectations which follow this path like an underground stream.

Even if it is true that in analysis there are no desires about the temporality of the treatment, it is also true that feeling *out of time* for a treatment cannot fail to present itself in a problematic way, prompting several questions:

- Will the patient be *in time* for treatment and will it be *their time*?
- Will the analyst be in the *patient's time*, in their various times: historical, psychic, biological, synchronous, or diachronous?
- Will the analyst be able to stay in the patient's *counter-time*?
- And, before being analysts, do we as humans know how to stay *in time* and in its complexities?
- And can we also stay *in the time* of war and self-destructive damage to the climate, retaining our faith in a Science which, as Carlo Rovelli reminds us,[6] despite its deficiencies, can still give us some directions?
- Do we humans also know how to stay in that atemporality of literature and poetry, art and philosophy, described by Anne Denis, and in the timelessness of the unconscious, which is like an untouched, always inexhaustible reservoir, a "further" that is always available if we can reach out a hand to it?

It seems clear to me that writing does not give answers but renews questions which nevertheless try to identify an integrated direction in relation to space-time, a direction which confronts the solitude of isolation with the solitude of thought.

Because boundaries do not isolate, but define.

We are asked to make a synergic effort that may positively contaminate the possibilities of the future.

No longer Hegelian men on horseback giving the go-ahead to thought and history, but men on foot who, by land and sea, may construct new collective viewpoints, even if we will be walking for a long time to come.

Notes

1 Author's translation: "I have just started, and finished, writing a long book."

2 My italics. In the original French Anne Denis says, "*Cette atemporalité est à distinguer de l'intemporalité de l'inconscient.*" She is using the Greek prefix *a-* to indicate an active negation and the Latin prefix *in-* to indicate an absence. (*Intemporalité* is translated here as "timelessness," echoing Strachey's translation of Freud's *Zeitlosigkeit* in the *SE*.) Linguistically the two terms may be seen as equivalent, but for the purposes of reflecting on the nature of time in the unconscious, an epistemological distinction can be made between them.
"Atemporalité" evokes not so much an unconscious without time as an unconscious opposed to the linearity of existential time. This contraposition also justifies re-significations in *après-coup* – i.e., meanings which emerge at a temporal distance in linear terms (*nachträglich*) and yet serve psychically to give sense to something that occurred before but remained enigmatic.
By contrast, "intemporalité" (timelessness) means a condition in which time is absent, and even space-time as a whole may be annulled, as astrophysics demonstrates with the theory of time, space, and matter collapsing in black holes.
See Einstein A., *Zur allgemeinen Relativitätstheorie*. Sitzungsberichte der Königlich Preußischen Akademie der Wissenschaften, 1915 (in English in Lorentz H.A. et al., *The Principle of Relativity: A Collection of Original Memoirs on the Special and General Theory of Relativity*, 1952). Also Schwarzschild K., *On the Gravitational Field of a Sphere of Incompressible Fluid according to Einstein's Theory*, 1916; and Rovelli C., *White Holes: Inside the Horizon*, 2023.

3 My italics.

4 Author's translation.

5 Author's translation.

6 Rovelli C., *Reality Is not What It Seems*, 2014. And Rovelli C., *There Are Places in the World Where Rules Are Less Important Than Kindness*, 2018.

AFTERWORD

Antonio Prete

After reading a book and making mental notes "in the margin," one is no longer in the state pictured by Baudelaire at the start of "Le Voyage,"[1] that of the boy "*amoureux de cartes et d'estampes,*" looking at maps by lamplight, dreaming of a boundless world. The journey has been made beforehand by someone else, the author, who has recounted the colourful and adventurous story of their travels. And yet something of that childish desire for knowledge remains, nurtured by the imagination, in the book that lies open before our eyes depicting lands and boundaries but sprinkling them with questions, revealing new paths to follow in every line, possible trails to pursue each time we return to the book. Marina Breccia's psychoanalytic story leaves us with this opening onto a land where asking questions is the principle of knowledge. Knowledge about ourselves and our place in the world. Because time is the great theme of the essay, the reader is drawn into a narrative time which asks us to listen to it: as we listen we are presented with figures that initially are of course those of psychoanalysis, its language, its knowledge and practices, but set alongside the illumination and avenues suggested by other forms of knowledge, whether "disciplined" or otherwise. I am not using the orotund splendour of the word *discipline* because what is rightly happening here is a discipline putting its own knowledge into a dialogue with forms of knowledge that are quite distinct, or even remote from it: so anthropology is in dialogue with the history of religions and rituals, literature with forms of theory, natural science with physics, and physics with the areas of knowledge that concern the lived experience of the *bios*. Into this tightly dialogic theatre, the book brings the fire of its questions, a fire fed both by the experience of psychoanalytic practice and by a passion for reading. And in turn, it is as a reader that I note down, as if with a pencil, some brief reflections in the margin of my listening.

The musical title and its reverberation: *counter-time*, counterpoint, rhythmic contrast of the melodic line with other voices, the significance of the pause, attention to unaccented beats, the turning of attention towards that which lacks strength, the resonance of what does not appear: overall, *the presence of absence*. For me, this storyline, which in the present book is nourished by passages of reflection, analytic narratives, excursions into theory, musings on trauma and mourning and on their connection with all that is tragic in our era, summons me into a neighbouring realm of language, one that belongs to time in my work: poetry and its language. Which, of course, is not a definite or homogeneous time but one made of silences, of counter-times. First of all, the time in which poetry happens, the time of its writing, is an unexpected time: to fall into a poetic state, into an "*état de poésie*," as Paul Valéry[2] says, is to open oneself to a visitation by a time that comes from outside and from far away, a time that calls for a concentration which turns into an image, for a meditation that turns into word and rhythm and thus into time itself.

Then there is the time of silence which is the *prima materia* of poetic utterance. Here is a thought from the Spanish poet José Ángel Valente: "Un poema no existe si no se oye, ante que su palabra, su silencio" (*José Ángel Valente: Poesia completa*, 1979, p. 388) ["A poem does not exist if, before its word, its silence is not heard"].

Centrality of trauma, work of mourning, meditation on the tragic, on the forms of the tragic, from genocide to war, from the production of poverty to the destruction of nature, of its harmony: Marina Breccia's book traces reflective sequences onto this dark canvas which assails our time and needs to be transformed into a meticulous interrogation (such as *Le livre des questions* by Edmond Jabès, 1963, whose title indicates the seven sections into which he divides his wonderful meditation on the tragic time embodied in the word Auschwitz). In another of his books Jabès says, "One does not tell the story of Auschwitz, every word tells it." The poetry of Paul Celan – Jabès himself more than once told me about his encounters with Celan – has also gathered the era's great wound into words, has made the wounded word into the language of poetry, displaying the tragic in the rhythm of verse, the void that dwells in the blooming of the rose (*Die Niemandsrose*, 1963). The "listening to traumatic counter-time" that is brought into play in these pages is certainly linked with the listening which poetry transforms into words and with the listening that it asks from the reader.

Standing in the shadow of knowledge. In the shadow of other disciplines. That exercise is practised in this book, an exercise which is first of all a spiritual one needed by those who are searching, and any true search can use wonder as an impulse bringing the searcher closer to the threshold of discovery and knowledge. Standing in the shadow is also an exercise proper to those who translate. I gave the title *All'ombra dell'altra lingua* (2011) [In the shadow of the other language] to a book devoted to translation. Only in that shadow zone does the other's language, that of the author being translated, metamorphose into one's own language, preserving as far as possible the timbre and quality of the original while also attaining the status of a new form. In translation too there is an intriguing relationship in play, one that knots itself into the word and its silences: this is also an encounter with the other, in search of a new time which is the time of the new text in the new language, where the first language both is and is not present. In the analyst's work these figures of translation are put to work: in any case, it is in language and with language that a relationship turns into care: that is, the building of a new time.

This book has much to say about autobiography. About the contract between saying and listening involved in every autobiography, about the exploration of what in the self is hidden and the move to narrative, to the re-compositional light of narrative that this entails: interrogation of what has been salvaged from oblivion. And what we call writing – although it is often practised in realms that claim to be about *looking at the self* rather than *listening to it*, the description of the visible and of what happens and not a representation of one's own interiority – is always concerned with the self. Telling the story of the self, whether directly or entrusting it to masks or emblems or phantasies of the "I," initiates the movement in which the "you" can acquire shape and presence, the you as the beginning of recognition of the self.

To tell a story is to weave a meditation on big questions about the relationship between subjects and their relationship with the world – between intimacy and action, between the forms of desire and the encounter with the other, between the search for sense and the loss of sense, between the dream and the annulment of the possible dream: as is demonstrated in these pages by the attention paid to a great novel like Rousseau's *Julie: ou la nouvelle Héloise*. This novel brings us questions that belong to us, not only about the relationship between love and renunciation, between the dream of love and the construction of the everyday, between memory and the search for the new time: but also, and especially, about the nexus between friendship and love, and about the idea of a community that is still "to come."

Finally, standing on the brink of a dialogue, we must respond urgently, today, to a need strongly articulated in this book: to look for ways of making swift reparation for the perversely assiduous and methodical offence being inflicted on nature, on its integrity, on the way it shows itself to us, on its visible and invisible forms. The earth is hospitable. Mankind has repaid this hospitality by destroying, altering, consuming, exploiting, brutalising. The idea of a reparation, inseparable from the idea of regenerating relations between living creatures, must not abandon us at this time, which is also a tragic time.

Notes

1 "Le Voyage" is the final poem in the collection *Les Fleurs du Mal* by Charles Baudelaire, 1821–1867.

2 Paul Valéry, "Nécessité de la poésie," in *Œuvres*, 11, p. 1387, 1937.

Bibliography

Abelard P. (2003) *The Letters of Abelard and Heloise.* Penguin, Harmondsworth, 1132–1135.

Abraham K. (1909) *Dreams and Mythus.* Nabu Press, Charleston, Sud Carolina.

Abraham K. (1914) Traum und Mythus. Deutike, Leipzig.

Abraham K. (1927) *Selected Papers on Psychoanalysis.* Karnac, London, 1979.

Agamben G. (2009) *Nudities* (trans. D. Kishik, S. Pedatella). Stanford University Press, Stanford, 2011.

Alighieri D. (1968) *La divina commedia* (ed. N. Sapegno). La Nuova Italia, Florence.

Amartya S. (1999) *Development as Freedom.* Oxford University Press, Oxford.

Amati Sas S. (2020) *Ambiguità, conformismo e adattamento alla violenza sociale,* Franco Angeli, Milan.

Arendt H. (1963) *Eichmann in Jerusalem. A Report of the Banality of Evil.* Viking Press, NY.

Arendt H. (1966) *Eichmann in Jerusalem: A Report on the Banality of Evil.* Penguin, Harmondsworth, 2020.

Arens W. (1979) *The Man-Eating Myth: Anthropology and Anthropophagy.* Oxford University Press, Oxford.

Aristotle (1955) The poetics (trans. S.H. Butcher). *Aristotle's Theory of Poetry and Fine Art.* Dover, New Yrk.

Assoun P.L. (1984) *L'entendement Freudien: Logos et Ananké.* Gallimard, Paris.

Augustine of Hippo (2023) *On the Trinity* (Eng. trans. A. West Haddan). Dalcassian, Connecticut.

Aulagnier P. (1975) *The Violence of Interpretation: From Pictogram to Statement.* Brunner-Routledge, Hove, 2001.

Aulagnier P. (1979) *Les destins du plaisir.* PUF, Paris.

Aulagnier P. (1984) *L'apprent-historien et le maître- sorcier.* PUF, Paris.

Aulagnier P. (1984) *L'Apprenti historien et le maître sorcier: Du discours identifiant au discours délirant.* PUF, Paris.

Balestriere L. (2014) Intime e profondissime predilezioni.. Episodi 'psicotici', posizione diagnostica e transfert contattuale: in M. Balsamo (ed.), *a cura di, Momenti psicotici nella cura,* Franco Angeli, Milano.

Balsamo M., ed. (2014) *Momenti psicotici nella cura.* Franco Angeli, Milan.

Balsamo M., ed. (2015) *L'Autobiografia psicotica.* Franco Angeli, Milan.

Bastianini T., Bebe Tarantelli C., *et al,* eds. (2009) *L'impronta del trauma. Sui limiti della simbolizzazione.* Franco Angeli, Milan.

Bataille G. (1955) *Prehistoric Painting: Lascaux, or the Birth of Art.* Macmillan, London, 1980.

Bauman Z. (1999) *Liquid Modernity.* Polity, Cambridge, 2000.

Bengston V.P., Elder Jr G.H., Putney N.M. (2005) The life course perspective on aging: Linked lives, timing and history: in M.L. Johnson (ed.), *The Cambridge Handbook of Age and Aging.* Cambridge University Press, Cambridge.

Benvenuto S. (2011) La 'ripresa' estatica di Elvio Fachinelli: in N. Pirillo (ed.), *Elvio Fachinelli e la domanda della sfinge. Tra psicoanalisi e pratiche filosofiche.* Liguori, Naples.

Bible (1968) *The Jerusalem Bible.* Hodder and Stoughton, London.

Bion W. (1959) Attacks on linking. *International Journal of Psychoanalysis* 40 308–315.

Bion W. (1962) *Learning from Experience.* Karnac, London, 1984.

Bion W. (1965) *Transformations: Change from Learning to Growth.* Tavistock, London.

Bion W. (1967) *Second Thoughts.* Karnak, London.

Bion W. (1970) *Attention and Interpretation.* Tavistock, London.

Bion W. (1977–1983) *Bion in Rome.* The Estate of W.R. Bion, London.

Bion W. (1982) *The Long Weekend, 1879-1919: Part of a Life.* Routledge, Abingdon, 2019.

Bollas C. (1987) *The Shadow of the Object: Psychoanalysis of the Unthought Known.* Routledge, Abingdon, 2018.

Bonaminio V., Giannakoulas A., eds. (2016) *Il Pensiero di Winnicott.* Armando, Rome.

Bonnet H. (1952) *Reallexikon der ägyptischen Religionsgeschichte.* de Gruyter, Berlin, 2000.

Boris S. (1972) *Picnic sul ciglio della strada*. Mondadori, Milan, 1982.

Botella C., Botella S. (2001) La figurabilitè psychique. Delachaux et Niestlè Ed., Losanna.

Breccia M. (2006) *Le parole ritrovate,* Borla, Rome.

Breccia M. (2011) *Exilium. Oltre la Psicosi*. Franco Angeli, Milan.

Breccia M. (2015) Le trauma et le temps autobiographique. *Revue Belge de Psychanalyse* 65 65–72.

Breccia M. (2016) Terzo. Da Freud a Lacan e a Ogden incontrando Green. *Rivista di Psicoanalisi* (1) 171–174.

Breccia M. (2017) Le moteur de l'interprétation dans un binôme. *Revue Française de Psychanalyse* (5) 1473–1478.

Breccia M. (2018a) Identità eterogenea: Identità Personale ed Impersonale. *Rivista di Psicoanalisi* (4) 745–754.

Breccia M. (2018b) Rosă, Rosae, Rosae. Déclinaison-Construction-Déformation. *Revue Française de Psychanalyse* (5) 1321–1326.

Breccia M. (2020) Norma-follia-disseminazione. *Rivista di Psicoanalisi* (3) 753–760.

Breccia M., ed. (2014) *Narciso e gli Altri*. Alpes Italia, Rome.

Brecht B. (1940 [1962]) *Refugee Conversations*. Methuen, London, 2019.

Brezzi P. (1960) Il carattere e il significato della storia nel pensiero di Sant'Agostino. *Analisi e interpretazione di De Civitate Dei di Sant'Agostino*. Edizioni Agostiniane, Tolentino.

Bromberg P.M. (1998) *Standing in the Spaces: Essays on clinical process, trauma and dissociation*. Analytic Press, New Jersey.

Bromberg P.M. (2011) *The Shadow of the Tsunami and the Growth of the Relational Mind*. Routledge, Hove.

Camus A. (1947) *The Plague*. Penguin, Harmondsworth, 2002.

Capiaux J., Denis A. (2019) Anamorphoses et Atemporalité dans l'œuvre de Proust. *Revue Psychosomatique*, 1(55), 111–134.

Carroll L. (1865) *Alice's Adventures in Wonderland and Through the Looking-Glass*. Dent, London, 1954.

Castoriadis C. (1969) *Socialisme ou barbarie: Anthologie*. Acratie, Les Lilas.

Castoriadis C. (1975) *L'institution imaginaire de la société*. Points, Paris.

Castoriadis C. (1989) All'epoca del conformismo generalizzato: in Bellusci F., *Castoriadis: fine della filosofia? Tre saggi sulla crisi del pensiero e della politica*. Asterios, Trieste, 2012.

Castoriadis C. (1996) La crise du processus identificatoire. *La montée de l'insignifiance*. Le Seuil, Paris.

Castoriadis C. (1996) *La montée de l'insignifiance*. Le Seuil, Paris.

Celan P. (1963) *Die Niemandsrose: Gedichte*. S. Fischer Verlag, Frankfurt.

Chabert C. (1992) Piera Aulagnier: 'Se costruire un passé'. *Topique* (1) 113–127.

Chervet B. et al. (2018) Destins de l'autoérotisme. *Revue Française de Psychanalyse* (3) 609–717.

Chervet E. (2017) *Patient et Interprète: Le domaine intermédiaire: 77° Congrès des Psychanalystes de Langue Française.* Interpréter, Paris.

Chervet E., Donnet J.L., et al. (2015) Réflexions sur la Dramatisation. *Revue Française de Psychanalyse* (5) 1529–1534.

Chetrit-Vatine V. (2004) La personne de l'analyste ou un espace matricie: l pour M. E. *Revue Française de Psychanalyse* (5) 1751–1757.

Chetrit-Vatine V. (2012) *La séduction étique de la situation analytique: aux origines féminines /maternelles de la responsabilité pour l'autre.* PUF, Paris.

Chetrit-Vatine V. (2018) Toucher à la dimension d'infinité quand le sexuel est tout autant au rendez-vous. *Revue Française de Psychanalyse* (5) 1507–1512.

Chianese D. (2020) *Il vivente e il sacro.* Astrolabio, Rome.

Clottes J. (2008) *Cave Art.* Phaidon, London.

Conrad J. (1917) *The Shadow Line.* Folio Society, London, 2001.

Contardi R., Gaburri E., Vender S. (1993) *Fattori terapeutici nei gruppi e nelle istituzioni: in Koinos Quaderni.* Borla, Rome.

Corsa R. (2013) *Edoardo Weiss a Trieste con Freud.* Alpes Italia, Rome.

Costis A. (2012) Piera Aulagnier: esploratrice instancabile degli abissi originari: in P. Cupelloni (ed.), *Psicoanaliste. Il piacere di pensare.* Franco Angeli, Milan.

De Gubernatis A. (1912) *Storia dell'etnologia.* Biblioteca Nazionale Centrale di Firenze, Perugia.

de M'Uzan M. (1970) Le Même et l'identique. *Revue Française de Psychanalyse* 34 441–451, and in *Cliniques* 13(1) 24–38 2017.

de M'Uzan M. (1977) *De l'art à la mort.* Gallimard, Paris.

de M'Uzan M. (2005) *Aux confines de l'identité.* Gallimard, Paris.

De Martino E. (1958) *Morte e pianto rituale nel mondo antico: dal lamento pagano al pianto di Maria.* Bollati Boringhieri, Turin, 2000.

De Martino E. (1959) *Sud e magia.* Feltrinelli, Milan, 2002.

De Martino E. (1961) *La terra del rimorso. Contributo a una storia religiosa del Sud,* Il Saggiatore, Milan, 2015.

De Mijolla-Mellor S. (2015) Specificità dell'autobiografia del paranoico: in M. Balsamo (ed.), *L'Autobiografia psicotica.* Franco Angeli, Milan.

Deleuze G. (1962) *Nietzsche and Philosophy.* Continuum, London, 2006.

Deleuze G. (1968) *Difference and Repetition.* Continuum, London, 2014.

Delourmel C. (2016) Green: rapporti del setting analitico con la funzione metaforizzante della parola e i processi terziari: in M. Breccia (ed.), *Dossier di Note storiche-critiche: Terzietà., Rivista di Psicanalisi* (1) 191–205.

Denis A. (1995a) Temporality and modes of languages. *International Journal of Psychoanalysis* (5) 1109–1119.

Denis A. (1995b) Le présent. *Revue Française de Psychanalyse* (4) 1083–1091.

Derrida J., Roudinesco E. (2001) *De quoi demain... Dialogue.* Champs Flammarion, Paris.

Donnet J L. Cherve E. et al. (2015) La dramatisatio. Revue Française de Psychanalyse 5 1517–1550.

Donnet J.L., Chervet E. et al. (2015) Réflexions sur la Dramatisation. *Revue Française de Psychanalyse* (5) 1529–1534.

Donnet J-L. (2005) *La situation analysante.* PUF, Paris.

Donnet J-L. (2016a) *Dire ce qui vient: association libre et transfert.* PUF, Paris.

Donnet J-L. (2016b) L'agir de parole: in *Des psychanalystes en séance. Glossaire clinique de psychanalyse contemporaine. « Folio »,* Gallimard, Paris.

Egidi Morpurgo V. (2006) Perché l'uomo Mosè ci inquieta ancora? Freud, la psicoanalisi e l'antisemitismo. *Rivista di Psicoanalisi* (4) 1087–1106.

Egidi Morpurgo V. (2007) Etica della responsabilità in Psicoanalisi nel dopo-Auschwitz. *Rivista di Psicoanalisi* (2) 515–527.

Egidi Morpurgo V. (2019) Di che cosa parliamo quando parliamo di etica della psicoanalisi? In e-book *Etica, Identità, Qualità. Scientific Training Day – Rome 12-13 October 2019.*

Einstein A. (1915) *Zur allgemeinen Relativitätstheorie.* Sitzungsberichte der Königlich Preußischen Akademie der Wissenschaften, Berlin. (In English in Lorentz H. A., Einstein A. et al. *The Principle of Relativity: A Collection of Original Memoirs on the Special and General Theory of Relativity.* Mineola, Dover, 1952).

Elder G.H. Jr. (1984) Perspectives on the life course: in G.H. Elder Jr (ed.), *Life Course Dynamics. Trajectories and Transitions. 1968-1980.* Cornell University Press, Ithaca, New York.

Elder G.H., Jr. (1994) Time, human agency, and social change: Perspectives on the life course. *Social Psychology Quarterly* (57) 4–15.

Elder G.H., Jr. (2000) The life course: in E.F. Borgatta, R.J.V. Montgomery (eds.), *Encyclopedia of Sociology* (2nd ed). Macmillan, New York.

Erikson E. (1950) *Childhood and Society.* W.W. Norton & Co, New York.

Esposito R. (2018) *Politica e negazione. Per una filosofiaaffermativa.* Einaudi, Turin.

Euripides. (438 a.C) *Alcestis and Other Plays.* Penguin, Harmondsworth, 1953.

Fachinelli E. (1964) Nuovo significato del disegno e recupero magico del passato nell'opera di un'artista psicotica. *Archivio di psicologia, neurologia e psichiatria* 25(1) 27–50, Vita e pensiero, Milan.

Fachinelli E. (1974) *Il bambino dalle uova d'oro.* Feltrinelli, Milan.

Ferenczi S. (1929) Theunwelcome child and his death-instinct. *International Journal of Psychoanalysis* 10 125–129.

Ferenczi S. (1933) Confusion of the tongues between adults and the child (The Language of Tenderness and of Passion). *International Journal of Psychoanalysis* 30 225–230, 1949.

Ferenczi S., Rank O. (1924) *The Development of Psycho-Analysis*, International Universities Press, Madison, CT, 1986.

Filoramo G. (2018) *Il grande racconto delle Religioni.* Il Mulino, Bologna.

France A. (1914) La révolte des anges. *OEuvres Complètes Illustrées*, Calmann-Lévi Éditeurs, Paris, 1930.

Francis of Assisi. *Cantico delle creature.* Cittadella Editrice, Assisi, 1982.

Frazer J. (1890) *The Golden Bough: A Study in Magic and Religion.* Oxford University Press, Oxford, 2009.

Frazer J.G. (1890) *The Golden Bough.* Macmillan and Co., London.

Freud S. (1887–1904) *The Complete Letters of Sigmund Freud to Wilhelm Fliess.* Belknap Press of Harvard University Press, Cambridge, MA and London, 1985.

Freud S. (1895a) *Draft K.* S.E. 1.

Freud S. (1895b) *Project for a Scientific Psychology.*S.E. 1.

Freud S. (1900) *The Interpretation of Dreams.* S.E. 4–5.

Freud S. (1905) *Three Essays on the Theory of Sexuality.* S.E. 7.

Freud S. (1910) *Psycho-Analytical Notes on an Autobiographical Account of a Case of Paranoia (The Schreber Case).* S.E. 12.

Freud S. (1913) *Totem and Taboo*, S. E. 13.

Freud S. (1914) *On Narcissism: An Introduction.* S.E. 14.

Freud S. (1915) *Mourning and Melancholia.* S.E 14.

Freud S. (1915a) *Mourning and Melancholia.* S.E. 14.

Freud S. (1915b) *Papers on Metapsychology.* S.E. 14.

Freud S. (1916) *On Transience.* S.E. 14.

Freud S. (1916–1917) *Introductory Lectures on Psycho-Analysis.* S.E. 15-16.

Freud S. (1919) *The Uncanny.* S.E. 17.

Freud S. (1920) *Beyond the Pleasure Principle.* S.E. 18.

Freud S. (1921) *Group Psychology and the Analysis of the Ego.* S.E. 18.

Freud S. (1924) *Neurosis and Psychosis.* S.E. 19.

Freud S. (1925a) *An Autobiographical Study.* S.E. 20.

Freud S. (1925b) *A Note on the 'Mystic Writing-Pad'.* S.E. 19.

Freud S. (1926) *Inhibitions, Symptoms and Anxiety.* S.E. 20.

Freud S. (1927) *The Future of an Illusion.* S.E. 21.

Freud S. (1929) *Civilization and its Discontents.* S.E. 21.

Freud S. (1933) *Why War?* S.E. 22.

Freud S. (1934–1938) *Moses and Monotheism: Three Essays.* S.E. 23.

Freud S. (1934–1938) Moses and Monotheism. Standard Edition XXIII.

Freud S. (1937a) *Analysis Terminable and Interminable.* S.E. 23.

Freud S. (1937b) *Constructions in Analysis.* S.E. 23.

Freud S. (1938) *An Outline of Psycho-Analysis.* S.E. 23.

Freud S., Abraham K. (2002) *The Complete Correspondence of Sigmund Freud and Karl Abraham, 1907-1925.* Karnak, London.

Freud S., Breuer J. (1893–1895) *Studies on Hysteria.* S.E. 2.

Freud S. (1923) *The Ego and the Id.* S.E. 19.

Gaburri E., Ambrosiano L. (2013) *Pensare con Freud.* Raffaello Cortina, Milan.

Gampel Y. (2006) *Rethinking Radioactive Transmission: The Riddle of Survival and Work in Situation of Political Violence.* Psicoanalisi e guerra: Il lavoro degli psicoanalisti in situazioni di conflitto. Pisa, 18.3.2006.

Gerson K. (1985) *Hard Choices.* University of California Press, Los Angeles.

Giaconia G., Racalbuto A. (1997) Circolo vizioso trauma-fantasma-trauma. *Rivista di Psicoanalisi* 43*(*4) 541–558.

Giddens A. (1995) *The Transformation of Intimacy.* Polity, Cambridge.

Gorz A. (1957) *The Traitor.* Verso, London, 1989.

Gorz A. (2006) *Letter to D: A Love Story.* Polity, Cambridge, 2009.

Green A. (1972) Notes sur les processus tertertiares: in Propedeutique. La Métapsychologie revisitée, Revue Française de Psychanalyse.

Green A. (1986) *On Private Madness.* Routledge, Abingdon, 2018.

Green A. (1993) *The Work of the Negative.* Free Association, London, 1999.

Green A. (1995) Note sui processi terziari. *Propedeutica: Metapsicologia rivisitata.* Borla, Rome, 2001.

Green A. (1998) *La Position phobique centrale*: in O. Jacob (ed.), La Pensée Clinique. Paris.

Green A. (2000) *Le Temps éclaté.* Edition de Minuit, Paris.

Green A. (2000) *Time in Psychoanalysis: Some Contradictory Aspects.* Free Association Press, London, 2002.

Green A. (2002) *Key Ideas for a Contemporary Psychoanalysis.* Routledge, London, 2005.

Green A. (2003) *La folie privèe: Psychanalyse des cas-limites.* Gallimard, Paris.

Green A. (2005) *Key Ideas for a Contemporary Psychoanalysis.* Routledge, London.

Green A. (2012) La posizione fobica centrale. *Psicoanalisi* (1) 5–33.

Greenacre P. (1967) The influence of infantile trauma on genetic patterns: in S. S. Furst (ed.), *Psychic Trauma.* Basic Books, New York.

Greenacre P. (1973) The primal scene and the sense of reality. *Psychoanalysis* (2) 106–130.

Grossman V. (1980) *Life and Fate*. London, Harvill Press, 1995.

Guamán Poma de Ayala F. (1615) *Nueva episodio de la Crónica y Buen Gobierno-Atahualpa preso en Cajamarca*. Biblioteca Nacional Colección, Madrid.

Heidegger M. (1927) *Being and Time*. State University of New York Press, Albany, 2010.

Hesiod. (1973) *Works and Days*. Penguin, Harmondsworth.

Hitler A. (1925) *Mein Kampf*, M. Amann Ed., Munch.

Homer. (1990) *Iliad* (Eng. trans. R. Fagles). Viking Penguin, New York and London.

Huber F. (2019) *Promise Me You'll Shoot Yourself: the Downfall of Ordinary Germans in 1945*. London, Allen Lane.

Jabès E. (1963) *Le livre de questions*. Blanche Gallimard, Paris.

Jonas H. (1979) *The Imperative of Responsibility: In Search of an Ethics for the Technological Age*. University of Chicago Press, Chicago, 1984.

Jung C.G. (1912a) The psychology of the unconscious. *Collected Works of C. G. Jung: Volume 7 – Two Essays in Analytic Psychology*. Princeton University Press, New Jersey, 1992.

Jung C.G. (1912b) Symbols and Transformations of the Libido. *Collected Works of C. G. Jung: Volume 5 – Symbols of Transformation*. Princeton University Press, New Jersey, 1992.

Jung C.G. (1952) *Synchronicity: An Acausal Connecting Principle*. Routledge, London, 1985.

Jung C.G. (1961) *Memories, Dreams, Reflections*. Collins, London, 1967.

Kaës R. (2012) *Le Malêtre*. Dunod, Paris.

Kerr J.F., Wyllie A.H., Currie A.R. (1972) Apoptosis: A basic biological phenomenon with wide-ranging implications in tissue kinetics. *British Journal of Cancer* (26) 239–257.

Kertesz I. (1975) *Fatelessness*. Vintage, New York, 2017.

Khan M.M.R. (1974) *The Privacy of the Self*. Karnak, London, 1996.

Klein M. (1921-45) *Love, Guilt and Reparation*. Hogarth, London, 1975.

Klein M. (1957) *Envy and Gratitude and Other Works*. Hogarth, London, 1975.

Kris E. (1951) Ego psychology and interpretation in psychoanalytic therapy. *Psychoanalytic Quarterly* (1) 15–30.

Kris E. (1956) The recovery of childhood memories in psychoanalysis: in *The Psychoanalytic Study of the Child* (1) 54–88.

Kris E. (1975) *The Psychoanalytic Study of the Child*: vols. 1–25. Yale University Press, New Haven, CT.

Lacan J. (1955–56) *Le Séminaire, Livre III, Les Psychoses*. Seuil, Paris, 1973.

Lacan J. (1957) The instance of the letter in the unconscious, or reason since freud: in *Écrits: A Selection* (trans. B. Fink). W. W. Norton, New York, 2002.

Lacan J. (1957–58) *Le Séminaire, Livre V, Les Formations de l'inconscient.* Seuil, Paris, 1998.

Lacan J. (1960–61) *Le Séminaire, Livre VIII, Le Transfert.* Seuil, Paris, 2001.

Lacan J. (1966) La chose freudienne: in *L'évolution psychiatrique*, Janvier-Mars 1956, pp. 225–252.

Lacan J. (1971) Transference: The Seminar of Jaques Lacan Book VIII. Polity Press, Cambridge, 2017.

Lambotte M.C. (1993) *Le discours mélancolique.* Érès, Toulouse, 2012.

Lantenari V. (1983) *Festa, carisma, apocalisse,* Sellerio, Palermo.

Laplache J., Pontalis J.B. (1967) *Vocabulaire de la Psychanalyse.* PUF, Paris.

Laplanche J. (1992) Du transfert, sa provocation par l'analyste: in Flammarion (ed.), *Le Primat de l'autre en psychanalyse.* Flammarion, Paris, 1992.

Laplanche J., Pontalis J.B. (1967) *Vocabulaire de la Psychanalyse.* PUF ed., Paris.

Laplanche J., Pontalis J.B. (1968) Fantasy at the Origins of Sexuality. *International Journal of Psychoanalysis* (49) 1–18.

Laplanche J., Pontalis J.B. (1973) *The Language of Psycho-Analysis.* International Library of Psycho-Analysis, London.

Laplanche J., Pontalis J.B. (1985) *Fantasme originaire. Fantasmes des origines. Origines du fantasme.* Hachette, Paris.

Laplanche J., Pontalis J.B., Lagache D., Nicholson-Smith D. (1967) *The Language of Psycho-Analysis.* Routledge, London.

Lattanzi V. (2000) Azione rituale, simboli culturali e storia. *Gruppo e funzione analitica. Koinos* (1) 20–27.

Lemkin R. (1944) *Axis Rule in Occupied Europe: Laws of Occupation – Analysis of Government – Proposal for Redress.* Lawbook Exchange Ltd, USA and Canada.

Levi P. (1958) *Survival in Auschwitz. (Originally published in English as If This Is a Man.)* Simon and Schuster, New York, 1996.

Levi P. (1986) *The Drowned and the Saved.* Abacus, London, 2013.

Lévinas E. (1949) *En découvrant l'existence avec Husserl et Heidegger (selections in English appear in Discovering Existence with Husserl).* Northwestern University Press, Evanston, 1998.

Levinas E. (1961) *Etique et infini.* Dialogues avec Philippe Nemo. Hachette, Vanves, 2006.

Levinas E. (2006) *Etique et infini.* Dialogues avec Philippe Nemo. Hachette, Vanves.

Lingiardi V. (2012) *La confusione è precisa in amore*. Nottetempo, Milan.

Little M. (1990) *Psychotic Anxieties and Containment: A Personal Record of an Analysis with Winnicott*. Jason Aronson, Northvale NJ and London.

Lombardozzi A. (2015) *L'imperfezione dell'identità. Riflessioni tra psicoanalisi e antropologia*. Alpes Italia, Rome.

Lyotard J.F. (1979) *The Postmodern Condition: A Report on Knowledge*. Manchester University Press, Manchester, 1984.

Manzoni A. (1840) *The Betrothed* (Eng. trans. A. Colquhoun). Dent Dutton, London and New York, 1951.

Margolius Kovály H. (1986) *Under a Cruel Star: A Life in Prague (1941–1968)*. Plunkett Lake, Lexington MA, 2012.

Marion P. (2017) *Sexuality and Procreation in the Age of Biotechnology: Desire and its Discontents*. Routledge, Abingdon, 2021.

Martin-Cabré L.J. (2021) Trauma, tracce primitive, e transfert. Paper read at the Centro Psicoanalitico di Firenze during the seminar *La psicoanalisi nel trauma contemporaneo*, 21. 10. 2021.

Martin-Cabré L.J., ed. (2016) *Autenticità e reciprocità. Un dialogo con Ferenczi*. Franco Angeli, Milan.

Matot J.P. (2020) *Le Soi-Disséminé. Une perspectiveécosystémique et métapsychologique*. L'Harmattan, Paris.

Mecacci A. (2008) *Introduzione a Andy Warhol*. Laterza, Rome.

Merleau-Ponty M. (1945) *Phenomenology of Perception*. Routledge, London, 1962.

Merot P., ed. (2019) *Folies de la norme*. PUF, Paris.

Mocan M. (2014) Un cuore illuminato: in P. Canettieri, A. Punzi (eds.), *Dai pochi ai molti*. Viella, Rome.

Moen P., ed. (2003) *It's About Time: Couples and Careers*. Cornell University Press, Ithaca, NY.

Moen P., Elder Jr. G.H., Lüscher K., eds. (1995) *Examining Lives in Context: Perspectives on the Ecology of Human Development*. American Psychological Association.

Naquet P.V. (2005) *Gli assassini della memoria*. Viella, Rome, 2008.

Neri C. (2006) *Pensieri senza un pensatore*. Seminar held at the Centro di Psicologia Analitica di Roma, December 2006.

Niederland W.G. (1974) *The Schreber Case: Pschoanalytic Profile of a Paranoid Personality*. Routledge, London.

Niederland W.G. (1984) *The Schreber Case: Psychoanalytic Profile of a Paranoid Personality*. Routledge, London.

Nietzsche F. (1872) *The Birth of Tragedy: Or Hellenism and Pessimism* (trans. and ed. D. Smith) Oxford World's Classics, Oxford, 2000.

Nietzsche F. (1882) *The Gay Science* (ed. B. Williams). CUP, Cambridge, 2003.

Nietzsche F. (1883) *Thus Spoke Zarathustra*. Penguin, Harmondsworth, 1961.

Ogden T. (1999) 'The music of what happens' in poetry and psychoanalysis. *International Journal of Psychoanalysis* (1) 979–994.

Ogden T. (2005) *This Art of Psychoanalysis: Dreaming Undreamt Dreams and Interrupted Cries*. Routledge, Hove.

Panikkar R.A. (2007) *Divinità*. EMI Editori, Bologna.

Pearlin L.I. (1982) Discontinuities in the study of aging: in T. Hareven (ed.), *Transitions: The Family and the Life Course in Historical perspective*. The Academic Press, New York.

Pearlin L.I. (1983) Tensioni vitali e sofferenza psicologica negli adulti: in N.J. Smelser E.H. Erikson (eds.), *Amore e lavoro*. Rizzoli, Milan.

Phillips A., ed. (2011) *The Christopher Bollas Reader*. Routledge, London, 2011.

Pini A. (2002) *Omocidi. Gli omosessuali uccisi in Italia*. Stampa alternativa, Roma.

Pitré G. (1871–1913) *Biblioteca delle tradizioni popolari siciliane*. Lauriel, Palermo and Arnaldo Forni Editore, Bologna, 1981.

Pontalis J.B. (1997) *Entre le rêve et la douleur*, Gallimard, Paris.

Porciatti V, Ventura L. (2012) Retinal ganglion cell functional plasticity and optic neuropathy: A comprehensive model. *Journal of Neuro-Ophthalmology* (4) 354–358.

Prete A. (2011) *All'ombra dell'altra lingua*. Bollati Boringhieri, Turin.

Prete A. (2013) *Compassione. Storia di un sentimento*. Bollati Boringhieri, Turin.

Proust M (1927) *A la recherche du temps perdu*. Bibliothèque de la Pléiade, Paris, 2005.

Proust M. (1909) *Correspondance de Marcel Proust: Tome 1*. (ed. P. Kolb). Paris, Editions Plon, Paris, 1989.

Pulcini E. (1992) *J-J Rousseau: L'immaginario e la Morale: introduction to Rousseau J-J., Giulia e la nuova Eloisa*. BUR, Milan.

Ranft L., Leipzig M. (1728) *Diceria del vampiro. De masticatione Mortuorum in tumulis*. Associazione Libri Perduti, Rome, 2011.

Rank O. (1900) *Traum und Dichtung*, 1914-1922 in appendix of Freud S. Dreams interpretation.

Rank O. (1914-1922) *Trauma und Dichtung*: in S. Freud (ed.), Appendix of Dream Interpretation- Die Traumdeutung- 1900 S.E IV-V.

Rank O. (1924a) *The Trauma of Birth*. Martino Fine Books, Connecticut USA, 2010.

Rank O. (1924b) *Das Trauma dre Geburt*. International Psychoanalytischer Verlag, Wien, Zürich.

Rank O., Ferenczi S. (1925) *Devolopment of Psychoanalysis*. Martino Fine Books ed., Mansfield, Connecticut, 2012.

Remotti F. (2001) *Contro l'identità*. Bari, Laterza.

Rohr P., Fritzsch B. (1679) *Dissertatio Historico-Philosophica de Masticatione Mortuorum*. Bavarian Public Library, Munich Germany, digitised 2011.

Roth P. (1986) *The Counterlife*. Vintage, New York, 2005.

Roth P. (1988) *The Facts: A Novelist's Autobiography*. Vintage, New York, 2007.

Rousseau J.J. (1782) *The Confessions, Book IX*. Privately Printed for Memberss of the Aidus Society, London.

Rousseau J-J. (1752) *Narcisse ou l'amant de lui-même*. Desjonquères, Paris, 2008.

Rousseau J-J. (1761) *Julie, or the New Heloise*. Dartmouth College Press, Lebanon NH, 1997.

Roussillon R. (1999) *Agonie, clivage et symbolisation*. PUF, Paris.

Rovelli C. (2014) *Reality is not What it Seems*. Penguin, Harmondsworth, 2016.

Rovelli C. (2018) *There Are Places in the World Where Rules Are Less Important than Kindness*. Penguin, Harmondsworth, 2020.

Rovelli C. (2023) *White Holes: Inside the Horizon*. London, Allen Lane.

Ruffini F. (2017) *La "Quaestio disputata de unione verbi Incarnati*. Edizioni Studio Domenicani, Bologna, 2017.

Saba U. (1988) *Tutte le poesie*. (ed. A. Stara) Mondadori, Milan.

Saba U. (2001) *Tutte le prose*. (ed. A. Stara) Mondadori, Milan.

Sandler J., Fonagy P. (1997) *Recovered Memories of Abuse: True or False*. International Universities Press, Madison CT.

Saraceno C. (2019) Solidarietà e voyerismo emotivo: in *La Repubblica*, 24.08.2019.

Scarfone D. (2014) L'impassé, l'actualité de l'inconscient. *Revue française de Psychanalyse* (78) 1357–1428.

Schatzman M. (1973) *Soul Murder: Persecution in the Family*. Random House, London.

Schneider H. (1995) *The Bonfire of Berlin*. Vintage, London, 2006.

Schneider H. (1998) *Il piccolo Adolf non aveva le ciglia*. Rizzoli, Milan.

Schneider H. (2004) *L'usignolo dei Linke*. Adelphi, Milan.

Schreber D.P. (1903) *Memoirs of My Nervous Illness*. New York Review of Books, New York, 2000.

Schwarzschild K. (1916) *On the Gravitational Field of a Sphere of Incompressible Fluid According to Einstein's Theory.* Sitzungsberichte Preuss. Akad. Wiss., Berlin.

Segre L. (2005) *Sopravvissuta ad Auschwitz.* Edizioni Paoline, Rome.

Segre L., Palumbo D. (2018) *Fino a quando la mia stella brillerà.* Piemme, Rome.

Semerano G. (2001) *L'infinito: un equivoco millenario. Le antiche civiltà del Vicino Oriente e le origini del pensiero greco.* Bruno Mondadori, Milan.

Sen A.K. (2000) *Development as Freedom.* Oxford University Press, Oxford.

Settersen R. (2015) Relationships in time and the life course. The significance of linked lives. *Research in Human Development* (12) 217–223.

Shakespeare W. (1600) Hamlet: in *William Shakespeare: The Complete Works*, Collins, Glasgow, 1960.

Shakespeare W. (1605) Macbeth:in *William Shakespeare. The Complete Works*, Collins, Glasgow, 1960.

Simonicca A., Dei F. (1998) *Dalla storia delle religioni all'antropologia.* Argo, Rome.

Smelser N. (1983) Aspetti problematici nello studio del lavoro e dell'amore nell'età adulta: in N.J. Smelser, E.H. Erikson (eds.), *Amore e lavoro.* Rizzoli, Milan, 1983.

Stara A. (2004) *L'avventura del personaggio.* Le Monnier, Florence.

Stara A. (2014) Dell'insolenza dell'io. *Homo Fictus* nella cultura del narcisismo: inM. Breccia (ed.), *Narciso e gli Altri.* Alpes Italia, Rome.

Starobinski J. (1989) *The Living Eye.* Harvard, Cambridge, Mass.

Strindberg A. (1897) *The Inferno.* (Eng. trans.C. Field) Putnam, New York, 1913.

Strindberg A. (1897) *The Inferno.* (Italian trans.L. Codignola) Adelphi, Milan, 2012.

Svevo I. (1923) *The Confessions of Zeno.* (Eng. trans.B. de Zoete) riverrun, London, 2018.

Tamet J-Y. (2022) Emergences de l'objet: paper read at 82nd Congrès de Psychanalystes de Langue Française, *L'objet, l'autre*, Paris 2022.

Tausk V. (1916) On the psychology of the war deserter. *Psychoanalytic Quarterly* (38) 354–381, 1969.

Thuan Trinh Xuan. (2016) *La plénitude du vide.* Albin Michel, Paris.

Toschi P. (1921) *La poesia religiosa del popolo italiano.* Libreria Editrice Fiorentina: Biblioteca di Filosofia, Università di Padova, Padova.

Turillazzi Manfredi S. (1979) *La linea d'ombra delle psicoterapie.* Del Riccio, Florence.

Tustin F. (1978) Psychotic elements in the neurotic disorders of children. *Journal of Child Psychotherapy* (4) 5–17.

Valabrega J-P. (2001) Les notions de Pictogramme et de Potentialité-psychotique dans l'oeuvre de Piera Aulagnier. *Topique* (1) 119–122.

Valdrè R. (2015) *Sulla sublimazione. Un percorso del destino del desiderio nella teoria e nella cura.* Mimesis, Milan.

Valente J.A. (1979) *José Ángel Valente: Poesia completa.* Galaxia Gutenberg, Barcellona.

Valéry P. (1894) *Les Cahiers.* Gallimard, Paris, 1973.

Valéry P. (1957) *Nécessité de la poésie: in Œuvres, vol 11.* Gallimard, Paris.

Ventura Avanzinelli M. (2005) *Sterilità e fecondità delle donne bibliche.* University Press, Florence.

Vico G.B. (1990) Principi di Scienza Nuova: in A. Battistini (ed.), *Opere.* Mondadori, Milan.

Virgil (2009). *The Eclogues and Georgics.* Oxford World Classics, Oxford.

Weber M. (1919) The profession and vocation of politics: in *The Vocation Lectures.* Hackett, Indianapolis, 2004.

Weil E. (2000) Silence et latence. *Revue Française de Psychanalyse* (1) 169–179.

Weil E. (2016) Traces psychiques, mémoires cryptées et catastrophes historiques. *Revue Française de Psychanalyse* (2) 488–500.

Weil E. (2021) Lieux du traumatique, le genocide: le nouage collectif-individuel. Rapport in 80° Congrès des Psychanalystes de Langue Française Espace psychique. Lieux, inscriptions.

Williams J.E. (1965) *Stoner.* Vintage, New York, 2012.

Winnicott D.W. (1939–1968) *Psycho-Analytic Explorations.* (eds. C. Winnicott, R. Shepherd, M. Davis). Harvard University Press, Cambridge MA.

Winnicott D.W. (1960) The theory of the parent-infant relationship. *International Journal of Psychoanalysis* (41) 585–595.

Winnicott D.W. (1963) Fear of breakdown. *International Review of Psychoanalysis* (1) 103–107, 1974.

Winnicott D.W. (1965) *The Maturational Processes and the Facilitating Environment: Studies in the Theory of Emotional Development.* London: The Hogarth Press and the Institute of Psycho-Analysis. *The International Psycho-Analytical Library*, 64:1–276.

Winnicott D.W. (1971) *Playing and Reality.* London, Tavistock.

Zaltzman N. (2007) *L'esprit du mal.* Éd. de l'Olivier, Paris.

Zaltzman N., André J., et al. (2015) *Psyché anarchiste: Débattre avec Nathalie Zaltzman.* (Petite Bibliothèque do psychanalyse), PUF, Paris.

Filmografia in ordine di citazione (Filmography in order of citation)

Derszu Uzala, 1975, Akira Kurosawa.

I misteri di un'anima (Geheimnisse einer Seele), 1926, Georg Wilhelm Pabst.

Il figlio di Saul, 2015, Laszlo Nemes.

La dernière femme du premier train, 2014, Daniel Friedman, In raccolta *Shoah pour mémoire,* 5 DVD, EM.

Le Mystére Picasso, 1956, Henri-Georges Cluzot.

Yuth, 2015, Paolo Sorrentino. *Stalker*, Tarkowsky, 1979.

Index

www.ingramcontent.com/pod-product-compliance
Lightning Source LLC
Chambersburg PA
CBHW061120050826
49324CB00036B/569
* 9 7 8 1 0 4 1 1 3 5 1 3 5 *